Professional Communication in Speech-Language Pathology

How to Write, Talk, and Act Like a Clinician

A. Embry Burrus, MCD, CCC-SLP

Associate Clinical Professor
Department of Communication Disorders
Auburn University

William O. Haynes, Ph.D., CCC-SLP

Professor Emeritus
Department of Communication Disorders
Auburn University

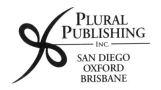

PLURAL
PUBLISHING
INC.

SAN DIEGO
OXFORD
BRISBANE

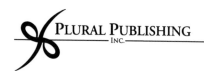

PLURAL PUBLISHING
INC.

5521 Ruffin Road
San Diego, CA 92123

e-mail: info@pluralpublishing.com
Web site: http://www.pluralpublishing.com

49 Bath Street
Abingdon, Oxfordshire OX14 1EA
United Kingdom

FSC
Mixed Sources
Product group from well-managed
forests and other controlled sources

Cert no. SW-COC-002283
www.fsc.org
© 1996 Forest Stewardship Council

Library of Congress Cataloging-in-Publication Data:

Burrus, A. Embry.
  Professional communication in speech-language pathology : how to write, talk, and act like a clinician / A. Embry Burrus and William O. Haynes.
      p. ; cm.
  Includes bibliographical references and index.
  ISBN-13: 978-1-59756-053-5 (alk. paper)
  ISBN-10: 1-59756-053-7 (alk. paper)
  1. Speech therapists. 2. Communication in medicine. 3. Interpersonal communication.
I. Haynes, William O. II. Title.
  [DNLM: 1. Speech-Language Pathology–education. 2. Clinical Competence. 3.
Interpersonal Relations. 4. Professional Practice. WL 18 B972p 2008]

  RC428.5.B84 2008
  616.85'506–dc22

                                                    2008042016

Contents

Preface

Let me tell you about Elizabeth, a composite of hundreds of undergraduate students who passed through our training program. Elizabeth was a sophomore who sat in the front row of my language acquisition class. She sported a pair of denim jeans with large holes in the knees and ragged edges around the ankles, a T-shirt that advertised an oyster bar in Pensacola, Florida, dark purple lipstick, and a diamond studded nose ring. Her hair was jet black and Gothic in style. I remember her as a warm and friendly student who wanted, more than anything else, to help children with autism. What occurred to me at the time, however, was the vast distance she needed to travel to make her dreams a reality. How could Elizabeth the Goth, who had no clue about the nature of professional service delivery, become Elizabeth the speech-language pathologist who works in a community clinic, school system, or medical facility? If Elizabeth did not get some instruction in professional appearance, professional demeanor, and professional communication before practicum started, her initial clinical experience would be like diving into a very cold pool of water. It is for this reason that most universities have a course with a title such as "Introduction to Clinical Practicum" that spells out in painful detail all of the rules, regulations, and behaviors associated with being a professional clinician. Make no mistake, the metamorphosis from student to professional clinician was not easy for Elizabeth, and she hit a few rough patches along the way. Fortunately, however, the end of Elizabeth's story is a happy one. Through 3 years of practicum experience in later undergraduate and graduate studies, she gradually learned to project herself as a professional and now is working as a certified speech-language pathologist in a large children's hospital. This book is designed to make the journey from student to clinician more predictable and a bit less onerous for students like Elizabeth.

Preparing a student for the clinical practicum experience has always been a challenge. The students come to us eager about embarking on a new and exciting profession. They have studied some of the disorders of communication in classes and seen videotapes of treatment sessions performed either by master clinicians in the field or more advanced graduate students. When the time for clinical practicum arrives, they are enthusiastic and worried about their first foray into a clinical relationship. Unfortunately, clinical work is one of those enterprises that almost all students enter with no practical experience. By our calculations, people in the speech-language pathology major have about 3 years to complete the transition from carefree undergraduate student to concerned clinical professional with a master's degree.

We asked ourselves many questions in planning this text: *Wouldn't it be nice if we could forewarn students about common pitfalls in the clinical practicum process, so these could be avoided? Would the student operate more efficiently in off-campus placements if we spent a little time introducing the nature of those settings before the student leaves the university environment? Would clinical reports be of higher quality if we gave examples and provided suggestions for writing and a list of common errors? Would the students be less anxious if we prepared them ahead of time with examples of the clinical documentation used in medical and school settings? Would the student be better able to verbally interact with clients, families, other professionals, and supervisors if we provided suggestions regarding professional verbal communication?* Clearly, we felt that the answers to our questions would no doubt be in the affirmative.

This textbook was designed to help beginning speech-language pathology students as they approach the clinical practicum experience. There are several major themes that weave their way through the text. First, we wanted to provide the student with a sense of professional demeanor common to speech-language pathologists. It is our view that such professionalism is largely communicated through our interactions. For instance, a person's behavior, written communications, and verbal communications are perceived by others as significant indices of professionalism. Actions can include such varied components as appearance, ethical behavior, decision making, planning clinical work, and nonverbal communication skills. Actions, as they say, often speak louder than words. Written communications range from various clinical reports to progress notes and professional correspondence. We project our professionalism every time we write any type of clinical documentation. Verbal communication with clients, families, other professionals, and supervisors is the means by which we provide information, obtain information, counsel, and solve problems related to clinical activity. Since the features of professional behavior, professional writing, and professional speaking are so important to defining a professional, we elected to name this book *Professional Communication in Speech-Language Pathology: How to Write, Talk, and Act Like a Clinician.*

A second theme of this book involves practicum settings. Since clinical practicum is different from any other experience these students have encountered, it is important to provide a road map of where they are headed in the process of learning to be a competent clinician. For this reason, we have chosen to discuss three practicum settings in almost every chapter: (a) university clinics, (b) medical settings, and (c) public school settings. The chapters provide examples of professional written communication that are unique to each type of workplace. Clinical documentation is similar yet different across these work settings and students should be aware of those similarities and differences before they experience an off-campus placement. But the information in this text goes beyond paperwork. For example, we discuss professional verbal communication in dealing with clients, families, other professionals, and supervisors across work settings as well.

A third component in almost every chapter is our delineation of proactive suggestions that are helpful to the student in navigating the various settings of clinical practicum. In this way, the book serves as a kind of survival guide to clinical practicum because we discuss common pitfalls across settings and ways to avoid them. If we expect students to perform well across different practicum experiences, then we should tell them how their behavior and documentation should change in these settings as compared to the university clinic. In many cases, it is as simple as just listing things to do and not do. Ironically, many of the pitfalls in practicum settings are caused by poor communication. Fortunately, it is also professional communication that plays a major role in solving practicum difficulties.

The final characteristic of this book is that we attempted to write it in a student-friendly style with copious examples and vignettes to help the student understand the material not only intellectually, but on an emotional level as well. Many books on clinical practicum are compilations of rules, references, regulations, and writing exercises that, while certainly important, are often difficult to digest. This book generally discusses most of these issues, but also illustrates them in a practical and interesting way. We hope the text can be useful as part of a course that introduces students to the exciting arena of clinical practicum.

SECTION I

Introduction to Professional Communication, Clinical Practicum Sites, and Ethics

1 The Nature of Professionalism and Professional Communication

INTRODUCTION

The field of speech-language pathology is one of the most respected of the helping professions. Speech-language pathologists (SLPs) work in a variety of settings with a cross-section of the population and a diverse group of related professionals. When we think of the word *professional*, what does this really mean? Webster's Dictionary defines *professional* as "[p]ertaining to a profession or to a calling; as professional studies, pursuits, duties, engagements; professional character or skill." The definition implies that there are certain characteristics of a professional that not only include duties (e.g., assessment and treatment in the case of the SLP), but also interactions (engagements) and personal attributes (character or skill.) Typically, a person knows if the treatment being received is professional and can easily distinguish unprofessional behavior on the part of a service provider. Yet explaining what it means to act as a professional may be as elusive as capturing lightning in a bottle. It is not difficult to recognize unprofessional demeanor, as illustrated by this account by Joseph Snyder, a businessman who is suffering from depression:

Dr. Murphy's address on Mimosa Street turned out to be an old hotel populated by unsavory looking characters who sat on the rickety front porch. I found Dr. Murphy in the telephone book under "professional counseling services" which I was seeking for my depression. I had to wake the desk clerk who directed me to room 112 and I knocked on the door. A loud voice from inside the room yelled "COME IN." I opened the door to reveal a middle-aged man sitting in a dilapidated recliner wearing an old Oriental bathrobe and sipping on an umbrella drink. Surrounding the chair were old newspapers and fast food containers that had been there for weeks. Upon seeing me he said, "What's up?" It was clear to me immediately that professionalism is not conferred on a person by a simple listing in the telephone book.

The extreme example above illustrates lack of professionalism on many levels. The next day, Joe Snyder tells us of his second attempt at finding help:

The entrance to Dr. Estrada's office was a stained glass doorway between two large potted palm trees. The waiting room was lit by bright sunlight, furnished with striped wing chairs and had mahogany tables containing carefully arranged magazines. Behind a counter sat a receptionist who wore a blue silk dress and a smile. I approached the receptionist and told her that I had a nine o'clock appointment with Dr. Estrada. She said, "Please have a seat in the waiting room. Dr. Estrada will be right with you." In about five minutes, Dr. Estrada appeared, shook my hand and said "I'm Dr. James Estrada and its nice to meet you Mr. Snyder." Then I was invited into Dr. Estrada's private office. It was a large, wood-paneled room that included a library of books and journals, several framed diplomas and licenses on the wall and a number of decorative plants. After we were seated, Dr. Estrada said "Lets get started by having you tell me what brings you in to see me today." As I began to tell my story, I could not help but think that this was the way it was supposed to be.

The overall difference between these two vignettes could be described in terms of physical appearances of the offices, demeanor of the office staff, and the language used by the psychologists. However, an overall discriminating variable between the two scenarios is the construct of professionalism. In one situation, professional behavior was lacking and in the other it was not. Again, we know professionalism when we see it, but it is difficult to exactly quantify. That is probably because being professional involves many variables that all interact in complex ways.

According to Brehm et al. (2006), the notion of professionalism is not monolithic and is in fact composed of multiple components. One component of professionalism includes professional parameters such as ethical and legal issues that guide many aspects of clinical practice. A second component of professionalism is professional behavior, which includes " . . . discipline-related knowledge and skills, appropriate relationships with clients and colleagues, and acceptable appearance and attitudes" (p. 1). The final ingredient in professionalism is " . . . responsibility to the profession and to oneself, clients, employers, and community" (p. 1). Thus, the combination of professional parameters, professional behavior, and professional responsibility form the core of professionalism in any field.

Although the scenarios at the beginning of this chapter came from the field of psychology, the various aspects of professionalism could have been illustrated using many different fields. The literature from many health-related disciplines is concerned with professionalism both at the level of training programs and in the clinical practice after graduation. For example, fields such as medicine (American Academy of Pediatrics, 2007), occupational therapy (Randolph, 2003), pharmacy (Hammer, Berger, & Beardsley, 2003), and nursing (Clooman, Davis, & Burnett, 1999) all view professionalism as a critical variable in clinical practice and in training programs. But it is not only in so-called "white collar" positions that professionalism is important. Even in jobs that are technically not "professional" we have certain standards of demeanor that are expected. For example, when you take your car in for repair you expect a certain degree of professionalism from the employees. We expect restaurant employees to behave professionally when serving customers. Professional behavior is an important part of every job from plumbing and carpentry to lawn maintenance and selling of automobiles. In all of these fields we expect the practitioners to have certain knowledge and skills that allow them to compe-

tently perform the job and we expect to be treated with respect. If these expectations are not met, people tend to not return for additional services.

It should be no surprise to students that professionalism is an important and critical component in the practice of speech-language pathology. When clients and other professionals deal with the SLP, there are certain expectations for professionalism. The general public expects an SLP to work in a physical setting that instills confidence in clients and represents the professional as someone to be respected as a clinician. The language we use with clients and people from other disciplines should be professional in tone and content. The reports we generate in the course of assessment and treatment of patients should reflect the professionalism of our field. Professionalism is not just about how clients and other disciplines perceive us; it is also about how it makes others feel about themselves. If you treat a client with professionalism, empathy, and respect, it will create an environment that is conducive to positive clinical change. Hegde and Davis (1995) discuss how professionalism manifests itself in SLP for practicum students:

> . . . general rules of professional behavior include punctuality in meeting clinical appointments and clinic deadlines, working cooperatively with office staff, supervisors, and other student clinicians, assuming responsibility for clinic equipment and clinic facilities, being well prepared for each clinical session, and maintaining appropriate dress and demeanor. Professional demeanor is one of the initial factors on which a student clinician is evaluated. Professional demeanor is a vague term, but refers to such behaviors as appearing confident in your abilities, communicating clearly and appropriately with the client and supervisor, presenting yourself as a mature adult, following prescribed rules and effectively utilizing clinical time. (p. 58)

You can see that professionalism is not only expected of seasoned clinicians but of clinicians in training as well. One objective of this book is to help students realize the importance of professionalism in becoming a SLP and how one's behavior, language, and writing are important factors in becoming a professional.

PROFESSIONAL COMMUNICATION

One common thread running through the concept of professionalism is the idea that it is demonstrated largely through various forms of communication. The physical properties of a clinical environment communicate important information about professionalism as illustrated in the psychology examples on the previous page. Nonverbal communication can indicate confidence and expertise as well as empathy for the client. Verbal communication with clients and other professionals can be a clear indication of a clinician's knowledge about the field, empathy, and ability to perform assessment and treatment activities. Finally, written communication (e.g., letters, reports, treatment plans, progress notes) represents the clinician to others when face-to-face interactions are not possible. The notion of communication is inseparable from the construct of professionalism. It is how professionalism manifests itself to clients and other professionals. Thus, it is not simply a coincidence that we have used the term *professional communication* in the title of this textbook. The term is very broad and includes both written as well as verbal interactions. Figure 1–1 shows examples of professional communication that represent the written and verbal modalities. Although we will be spending more time on the written forms of professional communication, it is important to touch on verbal communication as well. Let us spend a little time discussing the types of professional communication illustrated in Figure 1–1. In subsequent chapters of the present text we will be covering each of these areas in more detail.

PROFESSIONAL WRITTEN COMMUNICATION

Both students and professionals are required to generate professional documents related to evaluations, treatment planning, and treatment reporting. Figure 1–1 shows several important areas of professional written communication:

1. **Diagnostic reports:** These are clinical reports that summarize the results of an evaluation including standardized and nonstandardized testing of a client who has received a formal assessment of his communication abilities. The diagnostic report becomes part of a patient's clinical record and is often transmitted, with client permission, to other professionals. Our reports represent not only the student who wrote them, but the student's clinical supervisor and the facility (university, hospital, school system) that performed the assessment.

2. **Treatment plans:** Students in training are often required to develop written goals and procedures in the form of a treatment plan that is submitted to the clinical supervisor for review and approval. Students may also be asked to include rationales from theory or research for goal selection and the use of particular procedures in the treatment plan. The treatment plan should represent the result of considerable thought by the student after reviewing the case information, appropriate textbooks and class notes on the appropriate disorder, and discussions with the clinical supervisor.

3. **Treatment reports:** These reports are designed to summarize the progress of a client in a treatment program and address changes in client behavior on goals and objectives of therapy. These reports become part of a client's folder and serve to communicate the treatment approach and progress to other professionals or future students who will work with the case in subsequent semesters. For example, a client being seen in the university clinic may also be seen in the public schools and treatment reports are routinely sent to the SLP in the school system to make him aware of the client's progress at the university.

4. **Progress notes:** Progress notes are short synopses written on a daily or weekly basis in a patient's working folder or hospital chart to summarize short-term accomplishments of goals and objectives. These notes are read by other professionals in medical settings as a way of communicating client progress in many areas. The supervising physician will also keep track of patient progress by reading such notes.

5. **Professional correspondence:** These are letters written to referral sources, parents, family

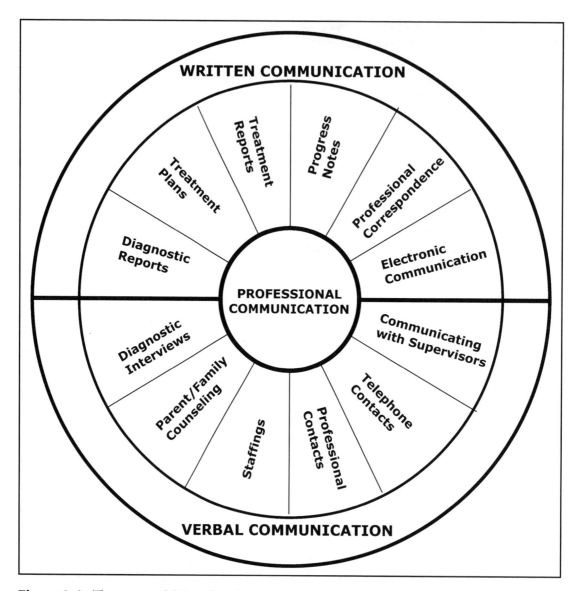

Figure 1–1. The two modalities of professional communication.

members or other professionals discussing general clinical matters or clinical issues related to a particular patient. Sometimes this correspondence is as simple as expressing appreciation for a referral from another professional. For instance, a physician may refer a patient with vocal nodules for voice therapy to the university clinic. It is always important to thank other professionals for referrals so that a good working relationship is maintained. You might also write a letter to a physician to whom you are referring a patient from the university clinic. There are many differ-

ent types of clinical correspondence and it is important that each be handled in a professional manner.

6. **Electronic communication:** The use of electronic mail or facsimile machines is sometimes used to relate clinical information to other professionals. Although we do not typically send reports via e-mail, it is important that any correspondence with other professionals or clients be done in as professional a manner as possible. It is not unusual for reports to be faxed between clinical settings, but as in any electronic commu-

nication, the importance of maintaining confidentiality of client information is paramount. For example, sending a report via fax relinquishes control over who receives it. There are some reports that temporary office workers should not have access to.

In all six areas mentioned above, the SLP is expected to adhere to specific professional guidelines regarding types of language used, protection of confidential information, and format requirements. The guidelines are similar across the six forms of professional written communication, but there are also subtle differences. These guidelines will be discussed in more detail in later chapters of the present textbook.

You might be asking yourself, "How difficult can it be to learn how to write all these different kinds of documents?" You may have been an excellent student in English composition, but unfortunately, clinical writing is quite different from generating a term paper or short story. In professional writing you will be expected to use professional terminology, write the document in the appropriate format, and employ very specific descriptions of a client's performance in reporting assessment or treatment results. You might be saying, "Why can't I just write it my way instead of using all these technical terms and strange formats?" Failure to understand the importance of clinical writing as a unique genre has led, on more than one occasion, to poor grades in clinical practicum. It is important for you to realize early on that clinical supervisors take professional written communication *very* seriously. Professional writing or reporting is *always* included on clinical practicum grading forms and students are evaluated on the punctuality of submitting paperwork, the quality of their professional writing, the completeness of the reports, and the appropriateness of the paperwork for the work setting. Ironically, although students are certain to be evaluated on these important facets of clinical ability, there is often little direct classroom teaching that focuses on professional writing. Textbooks most often devote a single chapter or part of a chapter to professional writing, and this is typically not enough exposure to prepare students for different types of reports (e.g., evaluation, treatment) or paperwork peculiar to a specific work setting (e.g.,

IEP/IFSP in schools, progress notes in medical settings, multidisciplinary reports, etc.).

How, then, do students learn professional writing skills if not in classes or textbook chapters? The reality is that students generally learn professional writing through the grim experience of generating a report for a clinical supervisor and then bearing witness to the supervisor figuratively "shredding" their work by slashing through the paragraphs with a red felt-tipped marker. In addition to the deleted utterances, the supervisor typically adds words and sometimes entire paragraphs with circles and arrows directing the student's attention even to the back of the page. Other supervisors merely make cryptic ciphers indicating that the student should "add more information," though not indicating how this should be done. This will lead to a second session of multicolored criticisms if the student cannot divine the intent of the supervisor. Students have also said that report writing style varies considerably by supervisor, and that what might be perfectly acceptable for one person may not be acceptable for another. An additional difficulty occurs when the student leaves the insulated setting of the university clinic for off-campus practicum. The student will soon learn that out there in the "real world," evaluation, treatment, and report writing are quite different from what goes on at the university. As such, students are buffeted about from one supervisor to another and one setting to another, and finally they "learn" professional writing through a process that involves much trial and error and some bruising of their egos. The present authors feel that professional writing is somewhat of a mystery to beginning students. We find it paradoxical that students are expected to learn professional writing largely through trial and error and with precious few resources that adequately address professional writing issues. This is precisely why we feel that a more proactive approach needs to be taken to professional writing in the form of a guidebook that is specifically directed to students in training. It is our hope that such a resource will demystify professional writing, illustrate appropriate formats used across work settings, discuss common errors that students tend to make, and show students examples of all the types of paperwork they will encounter at the upper undergraduate and graduate levels of their training. It is not possible to totally eliminate the frustrations associated with report writing for both students and supervisors because there is a certain amount of trial and error that *must* be experienced to learn this elusive craft. It is not necessary, however, to leave the entire process to chance. If we can provide explicit information in terms of report formats, typical writing errors, and professional language, the student can be more proactive and produce an initial effort that is closer to the desired target.

PROFESSIONAL VERBAL COMMUNICATION

The bottom portion of Figure 1–1 illustrates that professional communication is not confined to the written modality. There are many occasions on which students are expected to communicate verbally with parents, family members, or other professionals both in person and over the telephone. You might be thinking, "I already know how to talk to people. What is different about talking to people in a clinical setting?" Again, there is a certain professional demeanor and use of language that is expected in a clinical setting. There are certain terms to use, just as in clinical reports. There is even a "format" for what to talk about in certain situations. We will briefly mention the areas of verbal professional communication below:

1. **Diagnostic interviews:** No matter what type of client you see in a diagnostic evaluation, the interaction always begins with an interview. In the context of the diagnostic interview you will be interested in controlling the conversation so that you can obtain information, give information, and explain the assessment results to the client/family (Haynes & Pindzola, 2008). These interviews require organization, planning, and skill that few people innately possess, and prowess comes with practice. Later in the text we will talk more about professional communication in diagnostic interviews. For now, however, it is enough to realize that professional communication involves talking as well as writing.
2. **Parent/family counseling:** There are many occasions when we talk to parents and family members about treatment progress, referrals, or enlisting their help with the therapy program. Again, there are specific ways to communicate about such issues.
3. **Staffings:** In many work settings, a variety of professionals from different disciplines gather around a table together to discuss a particular client. For example, it would not be unusual to see a staffing that included an SLP, psychologist, classroom teacher, parent, and occupational therapist. Each professional contributes unique information to the staffing and is expected to communicate professionally. There are guidelines for professional communication in such settings and we will discuss these in later sections.
4. **Professional contacts:** In some cases the SLP will be asked to talk with physicians, physical therapists, radiologists, psychologists, teachers, special educators, and other professionals about a case. Although these are informal contacts, they still have the aura of professional communication.
5. **Telephone contacts:** Everything from scheduling cases for assessment and treatment to making referrals of a client to another professional often requires talking on the telephone. Again, professional verbal communication is critical.
6. **Communicating with supervisors:** As a student, you will have many opportunities to communicate with clinical supervisors, special education coordinators, directors of SLP in medical settings, principals of schools, and other people to whom you have to answer for your activities. Professional verbal communication is important in all of these situations. You may be explaining the progress of a particular case or lobbying for monetary support to purchase tests and materials. Professional verbal communication is a key ingredient.

SHARED COMPONENTS OF PROFESSIONAL WRITTEN AND VERBAL COMMUNICATION

Figure 1–2 shows some shared components of professional written and verbal communication. By shared components, we mean that certain commonalities

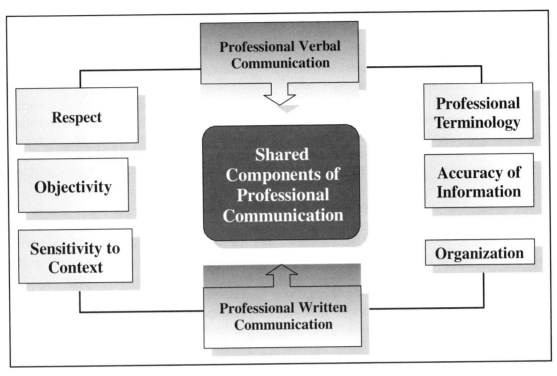

Figure 1–2. Shared components of profession written and verbal communication.

exist between the written and verbal expressions of professional communication. In many ways these components help to differentiate professional communication from a typical conversational chat. We will briefly discuss each of them below:

1. **Professional terminology:** In both verbal and written professional communication it is expected that appropriate terminology will be used by the SLP. We use terms such as *oral cavity* instead of *mouth* or *phonemes* instead of *sounds*. The SLP will discuss syntax, semantics, pragmatics, and morphology when talking about language. In both verbal and written interactions professional terms are appropriate to use, depending on the audience. As we will discuss later, the context of communication in terms of where you are talking and to whom you are talking is important to consider when using discipline-specific terminology.

2. **Accuracy of information:** It is assumed that any professional communication will contain accurate information, whether it is a verbal inter-

action or a clinical report. If a professional is asked how a child scored on a test, it would not be appropriate to say, "I think he scored in the 5th percentile, or maybe the 40th." If you can't remember the score, do not speculate. In a written report, we describe assessment and treatment information accurately using test scores and descriptions of behavior because we do not want to say something without reliable evidence. Professionals always double-check the scoring and reporting of test data to insure that it is accurate. There is typically a portion of a clinical report that allows a practitioner an opportunity to discuss "clinical impressions." This section of a report, however, is clearly demarcated from the parts of the writing that describe test scores and more objective information. Professional communication is highly concerned with accuracy.

3. **Organization:** Professional communication is usually orderly both in the written and verbal modalities. If you are part of a multidisciplinary staffing and are asked to talk about a child's language disorder and progress in treatment, the

other professionals present do not expect you to embark on an unorganized stream of consciousness rant about the client. They expect you to provide some background information, talk a bit about assessment, outline the treatment goals, and discuss progress in therapy. Even though you are talking, there is a basic organization that is expected from a professional. Obviously, in clinical reports, there is a format that is unique to the work setting that guides your writing. Again, it is not like writing a letter home to your family, but a highly organized summary of very specific information written in professional language. Thus, organization is part of both written and verbal professional communication.

4. **Respect:** One of the hallmarks of professional communication involves showing respect for the client, family, or other professional. This is not merely a courtesy, but is demanded by the codes of ethics of virtually every professional organization. We must treat patients, families, and other professionals with respect as an ethical proscription. This is why we usually refer to adult clients as "Mr. Smith" or "Mrs. Jones" rather than "Charlie" or "Edith." Certainly, as a clinical relationship develops we may refer to clients by their first names, but only when it is mutually agreeable and appropriate. Respect is also shown when we take into account the feelings and attitudes of others in the course of our interactions. We do not want to offend clients or other professionals with either our reports or verbal interactions. We show respect when we listen to the opinions of other professionals about our clients and when we listen to our patients as they tell us about their struggles. Respect is even shown in the quality of our physical facilities, the comfort of the chairs, and the reading material provided in our waiting rooms. After all, making patients wait in the squalor of a filthy, disorganized waiting room is a sign of disrespect to our clients. If we show up at the clinic in a T-shirt and jeans, we are saying to our clients that we do not think enough of them to present a professional appearance.

5. **Objectivity:** Part of professional communication, whether verbal or in writing, is that it is unbiased and reflects objective reality as much as possible. We assume that the professional SLP will gather appropriate information in an assessment and objectively interpret the data. Professional communication is not as much about a clinician's opinion as it is about evidence that can be documented. Professionals should never say something for which there is not adequate evidence or misrepresent the information that they are communicating. For instance, a clinician should not indicate that a child has cognitive limitations without the appropriate diagnosis. We would not want to indicate that a person has word retrieval difficulties without documenting this through assessment. For instance, if we said, "This child has behavior problems," it could be construed by the reader that he had actually been diagnosed with behavior disorder. It is much better to describe any behaviors that are of concern rather than provide inaccurate information.

6. **Sensitivity to context:** Contextual sensitivity affects professional communication in several ways. First, it is important to communicate in an appropriate way based on the setting in which the communication takes place. For example, in verbal communication in a hospital setting, certain words are used that are unique to that environment. One can use abbreviations such as *NICU*, *FIM scores*, *ADL*, *p.r.n.*, and *ROM*, and people in the medical setting will know what you are talking about. However, if you use these terms in the public school setting, teachers might not know what you mean. Conversely, in the school system you might use terms such as *Title I*, *Bloom's taxonomy*, *ESL*, *portfolio assessment*, and *IDEA*, which would be less understood in medical settings. At any rate, sensitivity to the context is an important influence on professional verbal communication. Context also has a large effect on professional written communication. For instance, the format for written reports and progress notes differs dramatically among university clinics, medical settings, and school environments. Your written communication must change depending on the context of the work setting. A second implication of sensitivity to context in professional communication concerns the person to whom you are talking or

writing. For example, parents are a very diverse group in terms of social status and educational level. You cannot explain the results of an evaluation the same way to a person with a graduate degree and another person with an eighth grade education, yet you have to do it professionally in both cases. In written communication, reports tend to be written in professional language and would not be understandable by some parents. In these cases we send a "parent-friendly" summary letter that tells them the critical information in the report. When talking to other professionals, we must discriminate which terminology people from other disciplines may and may not understand and adjust our conversation appropriately. Similarly, if we are sending a report, incorporating terms specific to our discipline might make our report less understandable to someone from occupational therapy. Thus, professional verbal and written communication must change with the context in which we are communicating, both in terms of the setting and the person to whom we are talking.

How do students learn about professional verbal communication? This is an interesting question because there are typically no specific courses that deal with the issue. Most students learn how to communicate professionally by modeling clinical supervisors and watching students who are further along in their training. Watching the behavior of an experienced clinician who is communicating professionally goes a long way toward teaching less experienced students how to act in a clinical role. In most cases, beginning students are not given the responsibility to independently interview clients, meet with other professionals, or counsel families. Students usually start by observing such activities during their required hours of observation. When students receive their first clinical assignments, they typically are asked to conduct certain parts of interviews, staffing presentations, or counseling efforts, but do not have independent responsibility. A student progressing through the training program is given a greater role in professional verbal communication and any missteps are pointed out after the interaction by the clinical supervisor. A good strategy for any student in training is to take advantage of every opportunity to observe your clinical faculty engaged in professional communication with clients, families, or representatives of other disciplines.

In the upcoming chapters we will be discussing both written and verbal communication in more detail to provide students with some general guidelines that will help you navigate your training program. As you will see in the next chapter, there is no one way to write reports, nor is there just one format for verbal interaction.

2 Learning as They Change the Rules: The Many Faces of Clinical Practicum

University Supervisor: "Always dress up when you are working with adults."

Hospital Supervisor: "You can wear scrubs to work."

University Supervisor: "Your report was not long enough and did not have sufficient detail."

Hospital Supervisor: "Your report was far too long."

University Practicum Student: "My client has been coming to the clinic for five years . . . we call him a 'lifer'."

Hospital Practicum Student: "We see our clients in acute care for only a couple of weeks."

University Supervisor: "Always take a detailed case history and put it in your report."

Hospital Supervisor: "Our only case history information is this checklist and a couple of lines in the chart written by the social worker."

University Supervisor: "Administer standardized tests in their entirety according to the instruction manual so you can compare the scores to norms."

Hospital Supervisor: "We rarely give a complete standardized test. We have taken tasks from many tests and made up our own assessment protocol."

University Practicum Student: "We always have to remember to shred copies of our reports for confidentiality reasons."

Hospital Practicum Student: "We have gone paperless at the hospital and I use a laptop to enter client data."

University Practicum Student: "I got graded down because I didn't develop a home program for my client."

Skilled Nursing Practicum Student: "My clients will never go home, and no one comes to visit them."

School Practicum Student: "We rarely see parents, except at IEP meetings once a year."

University Practicum Student: "My last report was five pages long."

Hospital Practicum Student: "I got marked off because my report was more than a paragraph."

School Practicum Student: "Our school has a software program to generate IEPs."

University Practicum Student: "I see this little boy individually and it's hard to develop enough activities for an hour session to keep him busy."

School Practicum Student: "I work mostly with kids in groups for less than half an hour."

University Practicum Student: "I have five goals I'm working on with my client; one is eye contact."

Hospital Practicum Student: "I have to be very careful how I write goals so we can bill for services."

University Practicum Student: "I'm working with a kid who substitutes w/r."

School Practicum Student: "In my school, kids with /r/ problems don't qualify for services."

University Practicum Student: "The kid I work with had the chicken pox last week. I felt so sorry for him."

Skilled Nursing Practicum Student: "My clients die just as I get to know them."

INTRODUCTION

The title of this chapter suggests that students in communication sciences and disorders will be confronted with many changes. On the surface, the statements from students and supervisors in the above box might seem in diametrical opposition. How can a clinical practice be acceptable to one student or supervisor on one occasion and unacceptable on another? Why is there such diversity in everything including clients, administrative procedures, opinions of supervisors, paperwork requirements, and types of therapy? The different perspectives illustrated above would seem to be a recipe for cognitive dissonance in our practicum students. Is it all part of an insidious plot to drive you completely insane? How

can you be successful if the rules keep changing? Do not despair. We are here to help you.

If you are reading this book as part of your curriculum in Communication Sciences and Disorders, we would like to welcome you to an exciting, diverse, and challenging profession. Over many years of teaching in a university training program, we have seen scores of students who decided to major in speech-language pathology. We have watched with great interest as they passed through the various phases of the curriculum and emerged on the other end as competent professionals. Through their training we saw the wonder on their faces as they began to understand the marvelous process of communication and all of the disorders that can rob a person of these critical abilities. We watched their first tentative therapy sessions and then saw them come strutting back from their internship showing all the confidence of a seasoned veteran. Over the course of training, however, we also were witness to many looks of consternation, confusion, and frustration as these students approached specific transition points in their programs. Much of their disquiet revolved more around the practicum experience than the coursework. Classes, after so long, become easy to deal with and students accepted into graduate programs usually have well-developed strategies for classroom success. Clinical practice, however, is a different matter. Here you are, after all of those courses, actually working with someone for the first time. Let us assure you that everyone in this situation is uncertain, apprehensive, excited, and clueless. One of the things that make practicum so uncertain is that there is no one way to do it. If there were a magic formula for planning, executing, and reporting every disorder the same way, it would certainly be easier. But there are different types of clients, multiple disorders, varied supervisors, and diverse practicum settings, all of which make clinical work confusing to the novice therapist. Students have reported several specific sources of frustration with their practicum experiences over the years. First, they do not seem to understand how the university training program interfaces with other settings to form the overall practicum experience. Students do not seem to appreciate the "big picture" of why the university training program teaches certain things and why other settings may conduct business quite differently.

A second problem for students is making the adjustment between practicum settings as they go through clinical training. Each setting has a different type of caseload, physical characteristics, professionals, and requirements for clinical reporting. The student is buffeted between long narrative reports in the university clinic, chart notes in medical settings, and IEPs in school systems. Just when you reach a certain degree of comfort in one format, you are asked to perform therapy and clinical reporting in a completely different way. It is not that we are trying to drive you completely mad; there are logical reasons for these inconsistencies. Any accredited program in communication disorders must insure that you obtain practicum experiences across different types of clinical environments. Thus, it should not be

a surprise that you will be plucked from the comfortable venue of the university speech and hearing clinic and transplanted into a rehabilitation hospital in the space of just a semester. Your first reaction will no doubt be shock. Virtually everything is different, and even though you knew on some level that practicum sites would differ, you had no way to prepare yourself for such an abrupt transition. Our motivation behind writing this book was to help ease some of the transitions for students who are moved abruptly across different practicum settings. One of the most frustrating aspects of the changing terrain is the different paperwork requirements and professional behaviors that are required. We thought that if students could get a preview of the requirements across sites, the transitions would be a bit easier. That is why we have organized this book to some degree by work setting. So, if you are headed to a hospital next semester, check out the parts of the book that deal with reporting and behavior in medical settings. If you are assigned to a local elementary school, look at the sections devoted to educational settings. One thing is certain; each setting has its own unique culture and set of requirements for behavior and paperwork. Granted, you will not fully understand the nature of these things until you have spent a couple of weeks in a new practicum setting, but knowing a bit about what to expect will lessen your frustration and apprehension. The bulk of this book will be concerned with professional communication across work settings, but we will also provide some suggestions about how to survive as a practicum student in each workplace.

In the United States, there are approximately 250 training programs in SLP that are accredited by the American Speech-Language-Hearing Association (ASHA). Within the context of each of these programs, undergraduate and graduate level students must earn about 400 hours of supervised clinical practicum across at least three different clinical settings. This means that the student must gain experience in university clinics, hospitals, community clinics, schools, and rehabilitation facilities with a wide diversity of clients representing many different types of communication disorders. Across all of these practicum settings and types of clients, the student in training is expected to participate in a variety of professional communications, both verbal and written.

DIFFERENCES AMONG CLINICAL SETTINGS

As stated earlier, students will be expected to participate in practicum experiences across a variety of work settings before they earn their graduate degree. The three most common types of clinical environments that students will encounter are university clinics, medical settings (e.g., hospitals, rehabilitation centers, nursing homes), and public schools. When students are initially placed in each of these three types of settings, they instantly notice that there are significant differences among the environments in terms of clients, the pace of assessment/treatment, and paperwork requirements. We would like to take some time now to clarify a couple of misconceptions students often have about how these settings relate to one another. First of all, it is important to realize that each setting is unique and there is no way that a particular type of facility can substitute for a different type of operation. For example, the university setting is typically a community clinic and cannot operate as a school or hospital. There is no way we can place beds in a university clinic or do video studies of swallowing. Likewise, we cannot use the university to act as an elementary school for large groups of children with communication disorders. University clinic training acts as a sheltered environment for initial clinical experiences and is not meant to substitute for or emulate medical or educational placements. In fact, some training programs do not even have an on-campus clinic and students will have to get all of their training off-site.

As mentioned above, students are sent to off-campus sites to gain unique clinical experiences that are not available in a university clinic. Sometimes students will complain that they have not been given practicum experience in dealing with swallowing disorders at the university clinic and have engaged only in classroom study of the issues. When they go to a hospital, they have their first hands-on experience with dysphagia. Of course, that is exactly why they were sent to the medical placement: to obtain experience that is not available in the university clinic. That is a good thing, not a deficiency in the university training program. Secondly, no one type of setting is superior to another. The sites are merely different. Students sometimes come back to the university after an off-campus medical placement and tell us that the experiences they had in the training program do not reflect the "real world" of the hospital or rehabilitation center. Of course, these medical placements do not reflect the real world of the public schools either, and vice versa. Students often forget that the university training program has a goal of exposing them to the real world, and this is accomplished through off-campus placements and internship experiences. Thus, it is simply not accurate to say that the university does not reflect real world practices; it systematically provides students with exposure to such settings through practicum experiences. University training programs are neither better nor worse than other placements; they are just different. At the university we try to present all of the relevant information and we may not necessarily tailor it to a particular work setting. That part is done by the supervising professionals who are working in medical settings and school systems. There may be many scientifically supported approaches to assessment and treatment that are "ideal," and these may have to be modified to be appropriate in medical or school settings. Thus, students should not think of one setting as being wrong when there are simply different ways of approaching clinical work in each one.

Some of the differences among settings flow from regulatory agencies (e.g., ASHA, Medicare, Department of Education, etc.) and others stem from the "culture" of each work environment. Table 2–1 shows the differences in regulatory agencies that dictate how each setting operates. University training programs are run a particular way because ASHA accreditation hangs in the balance. Medical settings are hamstrung by federal and state regulations, Medicare/Medicaid regulations, and insurance companies. Educational settings have a myriad of federal and state regulations to abide by in conducting their business. Table 2–2 depicts some of the differences in clinical operation in terms of caseload, supervision, and reporting. Just considering these primal differences among work settings should help you to understand why your practicum experiences will change dramatically depending on where you are assigned. We will elaborate a bit more on each work setting in the following sections.

Table 2–1. Practicum Setting Comparison Chart: Regulatory Control

	University	*Medical*	*School*
ASHA Regulations	• Heavily regulated by ASHA • Must train knowledge and skills • Accreditation requirements • Professional practice standards	• Not regulated by ASHA • Only professional practice standards and code of ethics apply	• Not regulated by ASHA
Federal Medicare Regulations	• No Medicare regulations unless clinic is a Medicare provider	• Heavily regulated by Medicare for adult clients	• Not regulated by Medicare
Federal Medicaid Regulations	• No Medicaid regulations unless clinic is a Medicaid provider	• Heavily regulated by Medicaid for child clients	• Not all systems regulated by Medicaid unless they bill Medicaid
Federal Education Regulations	• No federal education regulations	• No federal education regulations	• Heavily regulated by federal Education Department
State Education Regulations	• No state education regulations	• No state education regulations	• Heavily regulated by state education department
Federal Hospital Regulations	• No federal hospital regulations	• Heavily regulated by national guidelines	• No federal hospital regulations
State Hospital Regulations	• No state hospital regulations	• Heavily regulated by state guidelines	• No state hospital regulations
Third Party Payer Influence (e.g., insurance companies)	• Some clients use third party payers • Some insurance carriers limit the amount and type of assessment/treatment paid for	• Insurance companies regulate number and length of sessions paid for • Insurance companies regulate types of treatment reimbursed • Assessment and treatment are often driven by administrative regulations for billable hours	• No third party payers

The University Setting

Figure 2-1 shows a university setting, depicted as a series of "ivory towers" surrounded by several pictures. We have the ubiquitous professor lecturing to a class and another picture of a classroom using multimedia. Another picture shows a student dragging himself to the classroom with questionable motivation. The picture of the hand helping the person up the stairway symbolizes the sheltered environment of the training program where academic and clinical faculty are there to assist you if you have difficulty. Books, of course, are part of the deal in a training program, and we are aware that your tendency will be to sell them, but try to resist it so you won't have

Table 2–2. Practicum Setting Comparison Chart: Clinical Operation

	University	*Medical*	*School*
Caseload Issues	• Total control of caseload • Caseload determined by number of students and faculty and availability of clinical facilities	• Typically large caseloads • Little control of caseload	• Typically large caseloads • Little control of caseload • Legal mandates to provide free services to all qualified children
Pressure to Earn Income for Clinic	• Clinic income not usually the basis for faculty salaries • Often have sliding fee scale where patients pay according to income level and family size	• Pressure to generate billable hours • Income may be used to pay salaries and benefits	• Treatment does not produce income because it is free
Time Limitations on Clinical Work	• No time limitations on length of evaluations or treatment sessions	• Limitation on amount of time that can be billed to Medicare or third party payers	• Limitation on assessment and treatment time imposed by large caseloads and local regulations
Reports and Paperwork	• Reports are typically designed to teach clinicians to provide complete, accurate information • Reports may be lengthy with room for narrative explanations of case history information and interpretation • Greatest opportunity for lengthy reports	• Reports are extremely brief and may be limited to checklists with few opportunities for narrative • Reports may be in electronic format in a paperless environment • Least opportunity for lengthy reports	• Reports may include narratives, test scores, or depending on the school system, a form with check boxes • Treatment reports are often IEPs • Moderate opportunity for lengthy reports

to buy them all back for your professional library. Graduation and receiving your diploma are obviously the main goals; you want to be a certified speech-language pathologist who graduated with a master's degree from an accredited program. Finally, the stadium represents some of the extracurricular activities that are part of college life. Enjoy your experience as a student, because as you reach the end of your training program, it begins to approximate the feeling of a "real job." In our program, for example, students finish their master's training with a full-time internship in some sort of medical or educational facility where they are working from 8:00 to 5:00 every day. Their major comment is usually that they are tired at the end of the day and are thankful they do not have to study for classes and take exam-

inations. These same students will graduate, do their clinical fellowship year (CFY), and then they will no longer be students at all, but professionals with jobs, mortgages, and car payments. And take our word for it, you will long for those days when you were a student with less responsibility and much more free time. It's all part of growing up. The pictures we selected in Figure 2–1 are certainly not representative of all the experiences you might have had at the university; they were selected to portray the ambiance of your time in college. You will see when we begin to discuss other practicum settings that the orbit of pictures circling the hospital and school building are quite different indeed. This is because each setting has its own culture, atmosphere, and mood.

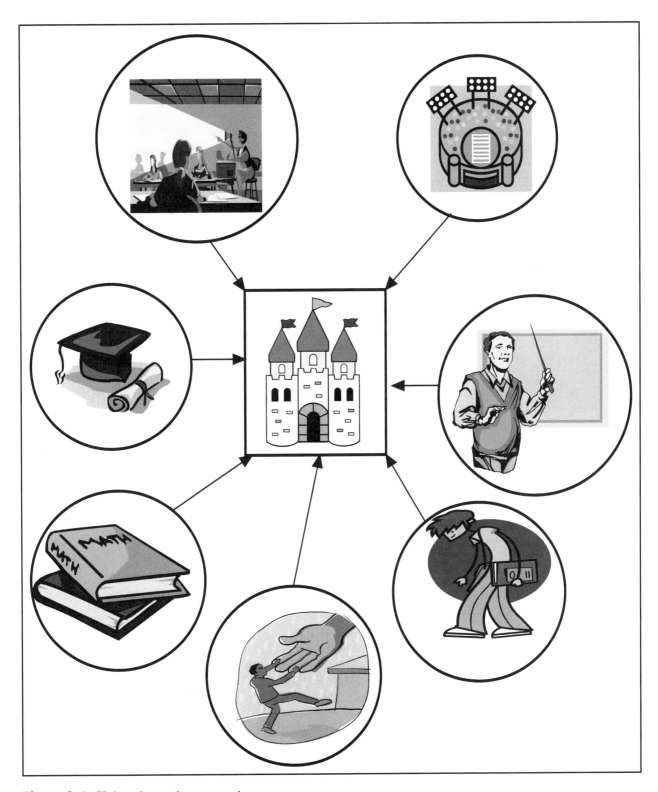

Figure 2–1. University settings are unique.

University training programs are largely designed to produce competent clinicians who are eligible for certification. Much of what goes on in the university training program is dictated by ASHA regulations and accreditation requirements. Figure 2–2 illustrates the flow of experiences in a university training program. Following are just some of the specific objectives of a university training program:

- Teaching a specific knowledge base in normal processes of communication (speech science, anatomy, physiology, phonetics, language acquisition).
- Teaching a specific knowledge base in disorders of communication involving phonology, language, voice, fluency, and swallowing. This knowledge base must transcend specific settings and represent the most current information and ideal standards of practice with particular disorders.
- Providing a scientific basis or rationale for assessment and treatment of communication disorders.
- Providing a sheltered environment for initial forays into clinical practice.
- Providing students constructive feedback on developing clinical skills.
- Coordinating additional practicum experiences in unique settings for experiences that are not

available in the university speech and hearing clinic.

University clinics typically have limited caseloads due to the regulations on supervision of students in training. Students must be supervised by a certified professional at least 25% of the time for treatment and 50% of the time for assessment. These requirements make it difficult for a university clinic to amass several hundred clients, due to the limitations of student clinicians and the constraint of having enough clinical supervisors. As a result, the caseloads in university clinics are small enough that clients can be offered assessment and treatment sessions that are longer than in other settings. For instance, clients might be seen for 1-hour sessions of therapy or have a 2-hour evaluation session. Longer sessions are desirable in the university setting because students must gain experience administering a variety of assessment and treatment techniques so they can demonstrate the knowledge and skills required for certification by ASHA. Think of how students and supervisors schedule time to plan for cases and engage in supervisory conferences to talk not only about the client's progress, but your developing skills as a clinician. This is a luxury that the university setting has, but other settings may not have due to large caseloads or restrictions of regulatory agencies and insurance

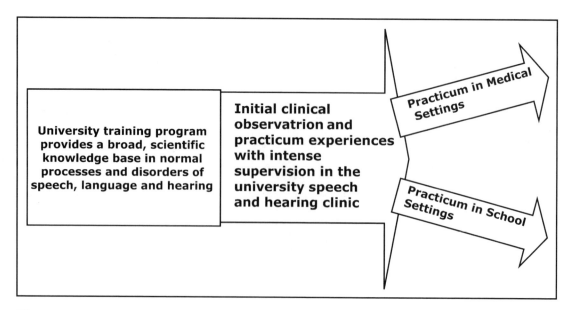

Figure 2–2. Progression of clinical training involving three settings.

companies that will only pay for limited treatment sessions. Most university clinics offer a sliding fee schedule or reduced prices for assessment and treatment. This also may not be seen in many other settings (private practice, hospital, etc.).

Another limitation of the university clinic is that this environment cannot recreate the ambience of a hospital or school system. It is difficult to prepare students in university clinics to deal with scenarios involving clients being taken from classrooms for therapy or adult patients who must travel by wheelchair from physical therapy to speech. With regard to report writing, most universities take the view that students in training should produce reports with the most complete data and narrative sections to illustrate the most that can be done with professional writing. At some point in your career, you may be asked to produce a formal report that will be used in a legal case or to establish eligibility for specific services on behalf of a client. In these cases, a simple checklist would not be the most appropriate type of report. There may be a need for explanation of the rationale for treatment and elucidation of how and why treatment targets have changed over time. Thus, university clinics are relatively sheltered environments in which students can be assigned limited numbers of clients and focus intently on the details of assessment, treatment planning, and the "long version" of clinical reporting. ASHA says that a student's initial practicum experiences should be in such a sheltered environment where time can be taken to learn some basics of clinical work prior to going to off-campus settings.

Easing the Transition into Clinical Practicum in the University Clinical Setting

As we said in Chapter 1, professionalism is all about communication. It is through communication that you project yourself as a professional whether it is verbally or in writing. It is important that you are proactive in approaching your clinical practicum and do some planning and preparation for the experience. If you are proactive, some of the fear of the unknown will be lessened and you will gain a certain amount of control over events. In some university clinics, you will have just completed undergraduate classes in the normal processes of speech, hearing,

and language and some of the disorders courses when you will have the opportunity to engage in clinical practicum. First, you will have the chance to observe assessment and treatment, and then you will be assigned a client or two of your own for which you take primary responsibility. Some of you might be in a training program that reserves all the cases for the graduate students. In that case, you can use our advice when you start clinical practicum on the graduate level. In most cases, however, undergraduate students have some opportunity to take responsibility for a case, typically in the areas of language or phonology. The case is usually a child, which limits your practicum experience to a specific group of clients. Assuming that you do engage in clinical practicum as an undergraduate, you will feel a distinct difference as you go from a student who takes classes to one who interacts with clients. You go from reading, listening to lectures, studying, and taking tests to planning, executing, and reporting clinical activities. Plus, there is a large increase in the expectation that you will act and communicate professionally. It is quite a jump from being a fairly anonymous student in a class of 30 to being on the spot as a clinical performer. So what advice can we give you to help ease the transition into clinical practicum and make it appear that your professionalism quotient is fairly high? We have some general suggestions:

1. **Look the part:** When you meet with your clinical practicum supervisor for the first time, make sure that you try to appear professional. You must remember that in many cases, your practicum supervisor may have never met you before, and if there was a prior meeting, it was probably in a classroom setting. In some instances, you may never have even had a conversation with one another. So it does not hurt to dress for success and come to your first meeting with a shiny new notebook in which to jot down important information. Remember that professionalism is communicated by your appearance, your demeanor, and the language you use.

2. **Be punctual:** When you have your first meeting, make certain that you are on time. It is extremely important once you begin clinical practicum to make sure you are on time for your

scheduled cases; your ability to be on time for a supervisory conference may be seen as a bellwether of your clinical responsibility to clients.

3. **Be prepared by reviewing your case:** When you go for your first supervisory conference, you no doubt will have been assigned a case with whom you will be working. It is always good form to have *extensively* studied the client's file from beginning to end. Do not just read the last report and omit the historical perspective. Supervisors will often ask beginning students to summarize the case as a way of beginning the first conference. If you are not prepared, you run the risk of being perceived as uninterested and unprofessional. Even if you are not asked to summarize the case, it is good policy to be as familiar with your client as possible. Usually, students tend to use the recommendations that were made in the most recent report as a template for planning their current approach to treatment. Although this is very logical, there is nothing wrong with having questions about the treatment approach that was recommended. If you find inconsistencies in the report, it is good to ask for clarification from the supervisor as to why they exist. For example, if the report is recommending the same goals and procedures used in the past semester, but the data show that the client made minimal progress, it would be logical to ask why you would want to spend the next 15 weeks doing what did not work in the past. You can make suggestions about applying concepts from your classroom work to the case as well. At the very least, you should ask questions about how a procedure was actually done in treatment sessions. It is almost impossible to recreate treatment tasks in a clinical report in sufficient detail to be replicated by a new clinician. So asking your supervisor, "Can you give me an example of how this task was actually done in a session?" is not inappropriate. If you can communicate that you are prepared for your first conference, your supervisor will tend to perceive you as having a high degree of professionalism.

4. **Be prepared by reviewing class notes:** Because you will be aware of the type of case you have been assigned, you will know the kind of disorder the client exhibits. For instance, if you

are assigned a child with a language disorder, you would be wise to review your notes from the courses you took in language acquisition and language disorders. If the client has specific symptoms or is in a particular stage of language development, you should especially refresh your memory regarding course information on this stage. Your supervisor might ask you a question such as, "What is the next thing to develop in a normal child at this stage of language acquisition?" It does nothing for your professional image if you shrug your shoulders and say, "I don't know." After all, you have taken several courses dealing with the topic and your inability to answer the question means that (a) you learned nothing from the course or (b) you did not prepare for the supervisory conference. Either of those reasons suggests a less than professional attitude.

5. **Talk with other students if possible:** If your client in the university clinic was seen the previous semester by a student who is still around, it is valuable to contact that clinician and chat about the case. You can gain much insight about the client, the treatment activities, the family, behavioral issues, room arrangement, and other information from a previous clinician. You can also get a preview of how the interaction was between the clinician and your new clinical supervisor. Sometimes the student will tell you some things to avoid: "Ms. Smith really hates it when you don't bring data to your conferences." Other advice might be on the positive side of the ledger: "She lets you use some of the therapy materials from her office." Get as much information as possible about your client, from any sources available to you.

6. **Use professional language:** As much as possible, try to use appropriate terminology when talking to your supervisor. For example, do not call phonemes "speech sounds" when you know the appropriate term.

7. **Define your responsibilities:** During the first conference make certain that you know what you are expected to do each week and throughout the semester. It goes without saying that you will be expected to be present for your therapy sessions. There are other meetings and responsibilities, however, that may not be as clear to you

initially. For instance, you will probably have to schedule a supervisory conference on a weekly basis to discuss your case and your developing clinical skills. If the meeting time is ongoing from week to week, block it out on your calendar. Make sure you know what is to be done during these conferences. For example, the supervisor may want you to bring treatment data on the client's goals to each meeting. If you do not bring it, there is little to talk about in the meeting and you are perceived as not meeting one of your professional obligations. Are you expected to generate a therapy plan each week? Are you expected to place a case summary devoid of identifying information in the observation room to assist observers? Do you have to write progress notes each week? Where are they and what is the format? Are you expected to transcribe language samples periodically to monitor progress? Is there a midterm progress report due on a particular date? When does treatment end and when is the final report due to the supervisor? What is your role in contacting other professionals working with your case (e.g., school system, psychologist) to coordinate programs or check on generalization? What is expected of you regarding parent counseling or devising a home program to assist in generalization? All of these questions are important for you to ask or clarify if they are not already addressed by your clinical supervisor. They show that you are interested in the case and professional in your involvement.

8. **Determine how you will be evaluated:** The interaction between you and your clinical supervisor has two major goals. First, both you and your supervisor want the client to be given appropriate services and make progress as a result. A second goal that is unique to training programs is that the supervisor wants to see your own clinical behavior change over time. It is important that you ask how and when you will be evaluated and how your grade in clinical practicum will be determined. In most cases, there are evaluation forms that your supervisor will share with you that show the behaviors and attributes she uses in grading your clinical competence. Sometimes supervisors leave notes after every session to provide feedback to stu-

dents. Some programs evaluate students midway through the semester and again at the end. However your supervisor provides feedback, it is critical that you get it often and early enough in the semester to make changes in your behavior. If you are not getting enough feedback, do not be shy about asking for it.

9. **Other expectations:** Be certain to clarify any expectations that go beyond the therapy session itself. For example, be familiar with clinic guidelines about infection control, disinfecting toys/materials, checking out of materials/tests, and returning the treatment room to its original condition for the next clinician. Also make sure you are aware of periodic meetings or staffings that you are expected to attend.

The Medical Setting

Figure 2–3 attempts to illustrate the mood of the medical setting. Note that it is considerably different from the university environment. Professionals wear specific clothing, in most cases "scrubs," which make everyone from a skilled surgeon to the maintenance personnel look like doctors. Patients, depending on their units, may be wearing hospital gowns or street clothes. Some patients are in bed and others travel by a variety of different conveyances such as wheelchairs, walkers, and canes. Some patients are hooked up to equipment such as IV stands or oxygen tanks. There is an obvious emphasis on infection control as evidenced by a smell of disinfectant and copious boxes of latex gloves. All of a sudden, you are working with other professionals from PT, OT, and nursing. You get the distinct feeling that you are not in Kansas anymore. In medical settings such as hospitals, rehabilitation centers, and skilled nursing facilities, there is a whole new set of regulatory influences on clinical practice. Whereas ASHA was the 800-pound gorilla in the university setting, medical environments are under no regulatory constraints from this organization. As indicated in Table 2–1, medical settings are mostly regulated by federal and state hospital guidelines, Medicare, Medicaid, and third party payers such as insurance companies. These influences will have a direct impact on what you do in practicum and paperwork associated with medical settings.

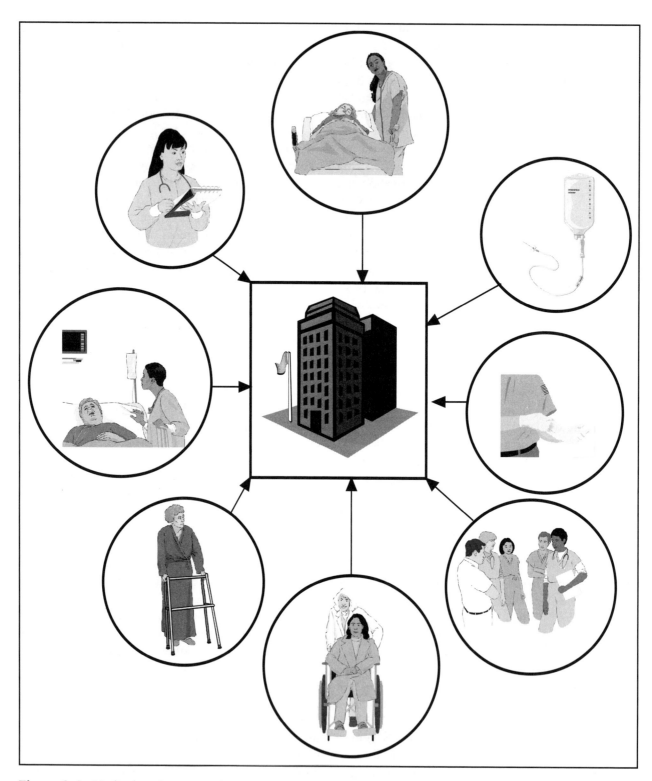

Figure 2–3. Medical settings are unique.

With regard to your training, medical settings have the following goals:

- Exposing students to varied caseloads of medically-based communication disorders in children and adults.
- Exposing students to the physical facilities typically seen in hospitals, rehabilitation centers, and skilled nursing residences.
- Exposing students to allied professionals (e.g., nurses, physical therapists, occupational therapists, physicians, radiologists) typically encountered in medical settings.
- Exposing students to the unique culture of medical settings with its attendant terminologies, equipment, and paperwork requirements.

When students go to a medical setting for the first time they are usually in a state of shock. First of all, the pace is considerably faster in medical settings because there are many more clients who are seen for shorter sessions as compared to the university clinic. Depending on the type of medical facility, a patient may only be seen for a week or two (acute care) and then be transferred to another facility for more long-term therapy (rehabilitation hospital). This is quite different from the university setting. In the hospital or rehabilitation environment, everyone is using terminologies that are unique to the medical setting, and students new to this environment are often intimidated by this unique language. Also, the student is interacting with other professionals in physical therapy, occupational therapy, respiratory therapy, and nursing, all of whom have their own jargon you have to learn and understand. Patients will be arriving in wheelchairs or using walkers or tripod canes. The patients may have just been to physical or occupational therapy and now must battle fatigue to participate in language treatment. Often, the clients the student dealt with in the university clinic were children with language and phonological disorders, and now the patients are adults who have neurogenically-based communication problems or dysphagia. There will probably be less time spent in supervisory conferences as compared to the university. In some cases, a facility will have a standard protocol for dealing with treatment or assessment plans, and very

little actual planning will be required of the student beyond how to implement the program. In some settings there may be a standard set of treatment materials in the form of a workbook that the student and client will use.

One of the biggest changes students see in medical settings is the different way of reporting assessment and treatment activity. The most noticeable difference is the brevity of reporting in medical settings. Students will do assessments in 30 minutes, and the "report" may only be a form that includes boxes to check with a few lines available for a narrative sentence or two. The patient's chart is a central point of communication in medical settings and the patient's status and progress must be summarized in only a few lines for other professionals to read. This is quite different from the lengthy narrative reports the student has written in university clinics. Students often complain that one of the most difficult things about professional reporting in the medical setting is learning how to communicate clinical results in a brief and economical format. What took an entire paragraph in a university report might only be communicated in a sentence or phrase in a patient's chart. It is not unusual for students who have completed a rotation in a medical setting to come strutting back into the university clinic in their scrubs and suggest that all of the time and detail spent on clinical reports in the training program were overkill and not reflective of the real world. It is important to remember, however, that before one can scale down information for a medical chart, she has to know what she is talking about. One cannot fully appreciate the elegance of a well-crafted, parsimonious phrase unless she understands exactly how the economical version really does reflect the reality of the patient's progress. We should always remember that checking boxes on an assessment form is often done at the expense of distorting the view of the patient.

Easing the Transition to Medical Practicum Settings

It is important to realize that when you arrive at a new practicum setting, you are not only representing yourself as a burgeoning professional, but you are also acting as a representative of your training program. Thus, it is critical that you think very carefully about the first impression you give to the professionals in your new practicum setting. Remember, the SLPs working in a hospital, rehabilitation center, or nursing facility are true professionals who have their own reputations to consider, as well as the reputation of their unit in the medical setting. Medical settings are divided into a host of different departments such as radiology, psychology, SLP, physical therapy, occupational therapy, and so on. Each unit has its departmental reputation to protect, and each professional working in the department is ultimately responsible for the actions of practicum students they supervise. If you create difficulties or act unprofessionally, it reflects not only on your immediate supervisor, but on that person's department and the university training program as well. So, like it or not, the pressure is on and the ball is in your court. You will remember that we promised to give you some good advice to ease the transition into different practicum settings, so in the next few sections, help is on the way.

We indicated earlier in the present chapter that a major purpose of this text is to assist students in developing professional attitudes and behaviors. One way of doing that is to think *proactively* as you move through your clinical practicum. We have tried to illustrate that one stumbling block in your practicum experience might be the differences you will encounter in the various types of work settings to which you are assigned. Knowing that you will have to make some adjustments in how you act and perform various tasks should be a first step to regaining control. It is important that you do some thinking and planning before you arrive at a strange practicum site. Be prepared to present yourself as a professional in training who has certain competencies but has come to the medical setting to learn more. Obviously, you are not coming to the hospital setting because you are a seasoned veteran who knows what to do. You have some knowledge from classes, and you might have even worked with some clients in the university clinic who have medically-related communication disorders. On the other hand, this may be your first experience with medical SLP. Whatever your situation, you can still make a good first impression on your new practicum supervisor(s). It is critical, however, that you not merely waltz into the hospital and say, "I'm here!" Adequate prepara-

tion on your part will make all the difference when meeting your supervisors for the first time. Following are some areas you might consider in planning your first visit to a new practicum site:

1. **Prepracticum visit:** We recommend that, instead of just showing up on your first scheduled day of practicum, you meet with your new practicum supervisor ahead of time. Actually, the medical facility may request this meeting before you do, but regardless of who makes the appointment, it is a good tactic to make a prepracticum visit. This shows you are interested, serious-minded, and professional.

2. **Orientation:** During your prepracticum visit you should ask about any orientation that will be provided by the facility for new practicum students. Again, your new supervisor may be planning to introduce this topic, but if she does not, you should ask. If the supervisor begins by telling you about a mandatory orientation meeting, you can say, "Good. That was one of the things I was going to ask about, and I'm so glad that an orientation is available."

3. **Being honest about your training:** Although practicum supervisors may see many students from university training programs, the students may have different levels of experience in medical SLP. It is important that you are honest about your coursework and practicum experiences at the university. If you have obvious gaps in your knowledge and experience, it is fine to tell your new supervisor what you feel comfortable with and in which areas you still have a lot to learn. It is especially important to communicate your interest in learning new things and that you appreciate the opportunity to learn as much as possible during your practicum experience.

4. **Learn names and the organizational structure:** Obviously, it is important for you to write down the names of any people you will be interacting with on a daily basis in the practicum placement. Do not be afraid to jot down those names because it is not unusual for you to meet many people during a visit including the SLP staff, people from other disciplines (physical therapy, occupational therapy, physicians, nurses), patients, hospital administrators, secretarial staff,

and other practicum students. It makes a good impression when you return if you can remember the names of people you met during your visit. Perhaps even more important than remembering names is figuring out the organizational structure of the facility in which you will be working. Like any organization, medical facilities have a power structure that is important to learn if you are going to be working there. For example, the SLP unit may be comprised of three SLPs, one of whom has administrative responsibility over the department. The speech-pathology unit may be part of a larger department that includes physical therapy, occupational therapy, respiratory therapy, and some other types of allied health professions. There is an administrator who oversees all of these different types of therapy and the SLP coordinator has to answer to this person. Our point here is that it is important for you to see where you are in the organizational arrangement of your medical facility and who is in charge at various levels. You never know when you will need to work with other departments and general offices such as risk management, security, or administrative offices. Your supervisor will tell you who is most important for you to know about while you are completing your practicum experience.

5. **Handouts:** It is appropriate for you to ask about the availability of any orientation handouts or brochures that cover policies and procedures of the facility in general and the SLP section in particular. Many practicum sites have informative manuals they have constructed just for practicum students to orient them to the setting. It is almost impossible for you to write down everything you are told in a prepracticum visit, so asking for a handout shows that you are interested in and serious about adhering to the rules and guidelines of the facility.

6. **Your schedule:** It is important to ask specific questions about your schedule such as when to arrive each day, where to report when you arrive, where to park, and when to leave. You cannot be punctual if you do not know your schedule. This would be a good time to have your supervisor describe a typical day you might experience, from start to finish. You should also ask about special events that will concern you (e.g., accreditation visits, hospital or department meetings).

7. **Responsibilities:** This is also a good time to ask about your responsibilities as a practicum student and how they might change as you gain more experience. You should ask about supervision in terms of how frequently it is provided and the opportunities for supervisory conferences regarding your caseload. Asking about the evaluation forms that will be used to grade your clinical work would also be appropriate at this time. It is possible that in some settings you will not see patients alone in the beginning. You may be observing or working with the facility SLP jointly at first. The supervisor can tell you how they work with practicum students, and you should be interested in this. It would be good to know that during a 15-week practicum experience, greater responsibility will gradually be shifted to you as you progress in the training.

8. **The facilities:** Ask for a tour of the facilities and where you will be seeing patients for assessment and treatment. Will you go to a dedicated room? Will you see some patients in their hospital room? Will you be working with groups? Where will group therapy be held?

9. **Transport:** Medical facilities have various regulations about transporting patients. Some patients in wheelchairs are often transported from one therapy to another by aides and sometimes by the person who just finished treating them (such as physical therapy). The point here is that you should be aware of what the conventions are in the facility and how patients get from one place to another. A major issue involves transferring patients from beds to wheelchairs, or vice versa. You should not do this without specific training because of possible injury to the patient or yourself. Find out the procedures that are used in your facility before you start working with patients, or else you could make a big mistake.

10. **Paperwork:** Because you will be required to produce many reports, notes, and other forms of paperwork, it is only logical that you should have the opportunity to look at examples of such output. In some cases, your supervisor will give you examples with identifying information deleted to protect confidentiality. In other cases, you

may be given an opportunity to study patient charts in the office. Whatever the case, it is good to familiarize yourself with the types of paperwork you will be asked to generate so that you can come closer to hitting the mark the first try.

11. **Confidentiality:** Ask about how patient confidentiality is handled at the facility. How is paperwork stored and secured? Are there secure computers available on which to do your reports? What disposal methods (shredding, erasing) are available for paperwork, electronic media, and audio/video tapes, and how is disposal accomplished?

The School Setting

In Figure 2–4 we try to capture some of the ambiance of the school setting. First of all, there are many children as opposed to the adults in medical placements. The professionals you deal with are regular education teachers, learning disabilities (LD) teachers, special educators, psychologists, special education coordinators, school administrators, and various support personnel. Children attend classes that focus on literacy, content areas of math, science, history, and social studies, and physical education. The classroom is an important milieu and you hear bells signaling the transition of one class to another or recess or lunch time. Placement in a school setting also has unique goals in your clinical training. Just as the university clinic and medical setting offer a special dimension to your education, school systems provide yet another facet to your developing skills. Some of the following are goals of the school setting related to your training:

- Exposing students to the varied caseload of the public schools ranging from preschool to adolescence. These caseloads can range from relatively simple disorders of articulation and language to very complex problems involving swallowing, augmentative communication, head injury, vocal disorders, and stuttering.
- Exposing students to the physical facilities typically seen in school settings from preschool programs to secondary schools.
- Exposing students to allied professionals (e.g., teachers, special educators, psychologists, aides,

administrators) typically encountered in the school setting.
- Exposing students to the culture of the educational setting with its attendant terminology, equipment, and paperwork requirements.

One thing that is immediately noticeable is that children are being seen for treatment in small groups, as well as individually. The school SLP may also do therapy within the classroom context and incorporate curriculum materials into treatment activities. As indicated in Table 1–1, schools are primarily regulated by federal and state departments of education. There are a series of laws that dictate how business is conducted in school systems ranging from the Individuals with Disabilities Education Act (IDEA) and No Child Left Behind (NCLB) to Section 504 of the Rehabilitation Act and the Americans with Disabilities Act (ADA). These guidelines will be discussed in later chapters; however, they are mentioned here to illustrate that schools are controlled by a myriad of legal guidelines coming from the state and federal government. Caseloads in the schools are typically high, which makes group therapy a more efficient way of providing services. School systems have very systematic procedures, just as medical facilities do for identifying clients and providing treatment. Specific forms, such as the *individualized education plan* (IEP), are standard fare in school systems, and we will talk more about these in a later chapter. Services are provided free of charge, which is a major difference from most other settings. Unfortunately, although the law says that every student should be provided adequate treatment, some school systems may be underfunded and not have enough personnel or facilities to service every child ideally. Other systems have state-of-the-art facilities, a full complement of highly qualified faculty, and small caseloads. Just as hospital settings vary in size, quality, and in terms of personnel, school systems do as well. Remember that school systems must service children from age 3 to 21, and many districts are providing assessment and treatment from birth onward. School systems use a variety of models to provide services including direct therapy, group therapy, consultative, center-based, and home-based programs. Thus, your practicum experience in the school environment can be

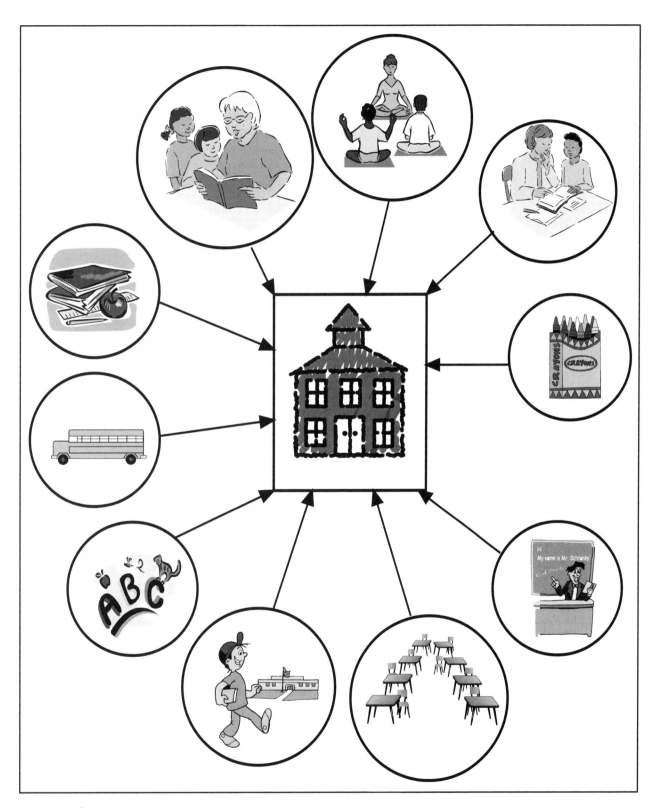

Figure 2–4. School settings are unique.

quite varied. In the past, the stereotype of a school system was that the caseload was largely made up of language and articulation cases. Today, schools represent one of the most diverse caseload environments available in clinical practice. It is not unusual to see children with head injury, unique syndromes, stuttering, voice disorders, cerebral palsy, autism, swallowing problems, and hearing impairments. There are children in the regular classroom who are on ventilators and who must use an augmentative communication device. Many of the children have been diagnosed with learning disabilities, attention deficit disorder, psychological difficulties, and behavior problems. Thus, the school environment is different from medical or university settings and this uniqueness is seen in assessment, treatment, reporting, and every other aspect of clinical work.

Easing the Transition to School Practicum Settings

Just as we urged you to be proactive in transitioning into your first practicum case in the university clinic and your introduction to a medical setting, we again suggest planning for your first visit to a school placement. Many of the principles we suggested for the other two settings also apply to practicum in the schools and we will not provide as much detail here:

1. **Prepracticum visit:** As in the medical setting, we recommend that you visit the school setting prior to your first day of practicum so that you can ask questions and receive instructions from your supervisor.
2. **Orientation:** In some school systems there will be an orientation provided for new practicum students. Be sure to ask about this and attend if it is offered.
3. **Be honest about your training:** In the school system you have a higher likelihood of working with children who have language and phonological disorders. This, in some ways, might be similar to your experience at the university clinic. You will have a larger comfort zone with these clients than you will have with medically oriented disorders in a hospital setting. Thus, you should feel a bit more comfortable in the school setting. Share with your practicum supervisor

the types of experiences you have had in the university clinic.

4. **Learn names and the organizational structure:** As in the medical setting, there will be many names for you to learn in the school placement: the SLP(s), school nurse, school psychologist, many regular classroom teachers, special education teachers, learning disabilities specialists, reading teachers, school administrators such as principals and assistant principals, a special education coordinator, and the secretarial staff. To compound this, you will often be assigned to multiple school buildings and so the names increase exponentially. The school organizational structure is both similar to and different from the medical setting. Schools tend to have a superintendent who oversees the entire school system. Each school is run administratively by a principal and assistant principal who control what happens in their building. SLP is typically under a special education coordinator who might oversee psychology, SLP, learning disabilities, special education, and reading disabilities. Thus, although you might be supervised by an SLP, you both may be ultimately responsible to the special education coordinator. In some large school systems there might actually be a SLP department composed of many SLPs, and one is designated as the head of the department. It just depends on the size of the school system. No matter where you are assigned, it is important to note where you fit into the organizational structure and to whom you are responsible.
5. **Handouts:** If the school system has any handouts on its policies, it is a good idea to obtain these and become familiar with them prior to your practicum. There may also be handouts generated by the SLP department that are designed for practicum students.
6. **Your schedule:** Like any work setting, there will be expectations regarding when you will arrive for work, when you can leave, and where you will go during the work day. School systems often have employees sign in and out of school buildings. You should ask specifically about your typical daily schedule and any special events (e.g., assemblies, staffings, IEP meetings) that you will be expected to attend.

7. **Responsibilities:** As in the medical setting, your supervisor might start you off with limited responsibilities and increase them as you gain more experience. You should ask about your initial responsibilities and how they are likely to change over time. This would be a good time to ask about the caseload you will be working with in terms of types of disorders, severity, and frequency of therapy. You should also ask if you are seeing the children individually, in groups, or in the classroom setting. This allows you to anticipate the types of activities you will need to prepare for treatment.

8. **Facilities:** You will want to know where you will be working with children in the school. Is there a dedicated speech pathology room? Is most of the treatment done in the classroom setting? Are you sharing a room with other professionals?

9. **Transport:** It is important to determine how the children will get to your treatment sessions. Will you go to the classroom and escort them to therapy? Will the children of a certain age be trusted to come to therapy by themselves? Will the teacher remind them?

10. **Paperwork:** The school system has unique paperwork compared to other settings. You will need to become familiar with IEPs and individual family service plans (IFSPs) and many other forms generated by the school system. It would be helpful if you could obtain example copies of such forms with identifying information removed so that you can approximate these models in your initial attempts at generating paperwork. We will discuss these in later chapters and have some examples in the appendices.

11. **Confidentiality:** In all settings you will be required to maintain confidentiality about your clients. You should ask about this issue in the school setting and determine how information is safeguarded and disposed of when no longer needed.

The purpose of this chapter was to introduce you to aspects of your upcoming clinical practicum that students rarely contemplate. Most students think of their practicum experience as a unified, seamless progression that is part of their clinical training. They rarely realize that there are unavoidable adjustments and bumps in the road that will make them question their abilities and the wisdom of those who designed their training program. Hopefully, this chapter has demonstrated to you that moving from one practicum site to another invariably means adjusting what you know and learning new approaches to old problems. The inevitability of having to make adjustments to different practicum settings allows you to anticipate these bumps in the road and take proactive steps to make the transition a bit more comfortable. The following chapters are designed to help you plan for different practicum placements and their attendant diverse environments, approaches to clinical work, and demands for professional communication.

3 Ethics, Confidentiality, and Safeguarding Clinical Communications

The field of speech-language pathology (SLP) is as diverse as it is dynamic and serves a large population of clients. This, in turn, makes speech pathology a public service. Those in the field recognize that the well-being of the people we serve comes first. To that end, confidentiality and safeguarding all information regarding our clients and patients are paramount.

Due to modern technology, public as well as private information is more accessible than ever before. As a result, identity theft and fraudulent use of confidential information has become commonplace. The need for guidelines to ensure the confidentiality of patients under any doctor's or specialist's care was not only recognized by the health care providers themselves but also by the federal government.

In 1996, President Bill Clinton signed the Health Information Portability and Accountability Act, or HIPAA, also known as Public Law 104-191. One of the provisions of HIPAA was to establish measures that ensure the security and privacy of health care information maintained by health care providers, both public and private.

How this relates to speech pathology encompasses many things. Private practices, hospitals, rehabilitation facilities, and long-term care facilities have many forms of communication that contain patient information. Most of this information is viewed by a diverse group of people involved in the patient's care. As a result, the speech-language pathologist may discuss patient and client issues with other relevant professionals on a daily basis. Referrals to other agencies may be made, resulting in information being passed via mail or electronically. It is imperative that the patient's information is protected so that abuse of any kind does not occur.

In addition, clients and caregivers have a legal right to read any report containing information about themselves or their family members (Family Educational Rights & Privacy Act of 1974, Public Law 93-380 [FERPA]). To this end, providers of SLP services must be accountable, not only in keeping accurate data regarding progress made in therapy, but in protecting the privacy of the clients they serve. Another fun fact about FERPA is how it impacts students. You would be surprised at how many calls your professors receive from concerned parents who want to know how you are doing in classes. According to the law, we cannot discuss student performance without your expressed permission. So, even though you might not have known about it, your privacy is being protected by the law. We hope, of course, that you are proud of your performance and share it with your parents, but it is your right to keep them in the dark, if you so desire.

ASHA CODE OF ETHICS

As professionals who are governed by a licensing board, we also have an ethical responsibility to our clients and patients. The American Speech-Language-Hearing Association (ASHA) has a code of ethics (ASHA, 2003) just as other professional organizations such as psychology, medicine, nursing, occupational therapy, education, and physical therapy prescribe ethical responsibilities of practitioners. We do not want to turn this chapter into a review of the entire Code of Ethics on issues such as practice, but we would like to mention certain ethical proscriptions that deal with professional communication.

Several portions of the ASHA Code of Ethics relate to the notions of professionalism and communication. We will quote these directly from the 2003 version of the Code of Ethics, and you should be able to see how they relate to *professionalism* and *communication* (ASHA, 2003):

- "Individuals shall not reveal, without authorization, any professional or personal information about the person served professionally, unless required by law to do so, or unless doing so is necessary to protect the welfare of the person or the community" (Principle of Ethics I, Rule L).
- "Individuals shall fully inform the persons they serve of the nature and possible effects of services rendered and products dispensed, and they shall inform participants in research about the possible effects of their participation in research conducted" (Principle of Ethics I, Rule F).
- "Individuals shall not guarantee the results of any treatment or procedure, directly or by implication . . . " (Principle of Ethics I, Rule H).
- "Individuals shall not misrepresent their credentials, competence, education, training, experience, or scholarly or research contributions" (Principle of Ethics III, Rule A).
- "Individuals shall not misrepresent diagnostic information, research, services rendered, or products dispensed . . . " (Principle of Ethics III, Rule D).
- "Individuals' statements to the public shall provide accurate information about the nature and management of communication disorders, about the professions, about professional services and about research and scholarly activities" (Principle of Ethics III, Rule E).
- "Individuals' statements to the public—advertising, announcing, and marketing their professional services, reporting research results, and promoting products—shall adhere to prevailing professional standards and shall not contain misrepresentations" (Principle of Ethics III, Rule F).
- "Individuals shall not engage in dishonesty, fraud, deceit, misrepresentation, sexual harassment, or any other form of conduct that adversely reflects on the professions or on the individual's fitness to serve persons professionally" (Principle of Ethics IV, Rule B).

- "Individuals' statements to colleagues about professional services, research results, and products shall adhere to prevailing professional standards and shall contain no misrepresentations" (Principle of Ethics IV, Rule F).

The word *professional* appears in almost all of these ethical guidelines. Note also that almost all of them also include the notion of "communication" either explicitly or implicitly. Many of the statements have a great deal to do with the idea that a SLP is expected to communicate with colleagues and patients accurately, in a professional manner, without misrepresenting his clinical practice. Even in our advertising we must meet "professional standards" and not place an advertisement as if we were selling used automobiles. It is no coincidence that announcements and advertising from many different professions (e.g., physicians, dentists, psychologists) all look similar. Thus, we hope you can see that our Code of Ethics places a great deal of emphasis on professional communication. In the next few sections we will zero in on the notion of confidentiality in both written and verbal professional communication across work settings.

THE UNIVERSITY SPEECH AND HEARING CLINIC

The university speech and hearing clinic will be your first foray into dealing with confidential clinical information and acting with a degree of professionalism. If you are not already aware of it, all of our clients deserve the right to privacy in seeking clinical services. Some of them take it quite seriously. We have worked with adult clients who have specifically requested that they not be observed by students in our training program. Although we would like to give students the opportunity to view all treatment sessions, we have to respect the rights of our clients to their privacy. Some clients request privacy only in the beginning of treatment, and then as they gain expertise in communication they are proud of their accomplishments and welcome observers.

George Adams was a retired history professor whose progressive Parkinson's disease essentially put a stop to his teaching career. He had an extremely tremulous voice and made uncontrolled upper body movements even sitting in a chair. Because Dr. Adams had taught at the university for 40 years, he came to the speech and hearing clinic for services. Because he had only retired a year ago he was concerned that some of his former students would still be around to see the ravages of his Parkinson's disease on his appearance and communication. He specifically requested that no students be allowed to observe his treatment sessions.

Michael (Michelle) Genrette had made a most drastic decision. He had decided to begin the process of sexual reassignment and become a woman. This very personal decision was not made lightly and Mr. Genrette had undergone extensive counseling from physicians and psychologists. As part of his transition from male to female he had to learn new vocal production patterns, nonverbal communication, and language structures common to women. Mr. Genrette was a faculty member at the university, and he had not yet shared his decision with coworkers or even some of his family members. Thus, it was important for the speech and hearing clinic staff to maintain confidentiality and not talk openly about this case. Mr. Genrette also requested that no one observe his treatment sessions.

The university training program is a veritable minefield of confidentiality issues. First of all, we generate reams of paperwork related to assessment, treatment, and student training. Second, much of this paperwork is handled on a daily basis by students who have never been responsible for protecting the personal privacy of clients. In the university speech clinic, sources of personal information include, but are not limited to:

- Daily notes and treatment plans
- Formal treatment reports
- Formal diagnostic reports
- Information on diskettes or flash drives used by students
- Electronic transmissions (faxes, e-mails, billing)
- Authorization forms signed by clients
- Therapy schedules
- Verbal discussions

Each of these will be discussed in more detail below.

Daily Notes and Treatment Plans

The progress note is a vital part of the SLP's daily routine. This information provides accountability for what takes place in a clinical session through data collection, assessment of a client's performance, and plans for future sessions. In the university clinic, the student writes a progress note after each session. These notes are often kept in a client file in the supervisor's office as part of the safeguarding procedure. The daily note may contain less personal information about the client, as the student may use a client's file number, date of birth, or initials as identifying information. However, if any form is discarded, it should be shredded rather than thrown away.

Formal Treatment Reports

The formal treatment report is a summary of client information and data collection usually for one semester. These reports include a great deal of personal information about a client such as name, date of birth, address, telephone number, referring physician, diagnosis, and so forth. It is important that this information is not handled casually and that the student or students who are working with this client do not leave these reports in public areas where anyone can read this confidential information.

Copy Confusion

Carmen Jones was in a hurry. Her treatment reports on five clients were due to be turned in to her supervisor in less than an hour. She needed to make three copies of each report for distribution to the client folder, parents, and the school system. Carmen found an open Xerox machine at the local copying store and placed each of her five reports in the feeder tray, pressing the appropriate buttons for three copies each. As the copies came out, Carmen paper-clipped them together in a pile and removed the original from the machine. When the last copy was done, she looked at her watch and realized that she only had 10 minutes to get to the clinic. As Carmen grabbed all her copies and rushed out the door, she was oblivious to the fact that the original from the last report she had copied remained in the document feeder. The next person to use that machine would have a golden opportunity to learn about Tyrone Walker, an elementary school student with autism whose mother places a high value on privacy.

Formal Diagnostic Reports

Just as with the formal treatment report, the diagnostic report also contains a great deal of personal information about a client. In fact, the diagnostic report is likely to contain the most personal data of any of our professional communications. By their very nature, the diagnostic report contains a plethora of historical information, not only about the client, but the family as well. So, if a child exhibits behavior problems, bed-wetting or thumb-sucking, it is all laid out in the case history. If a child has developed dysfluencies since his parents' divorce, it is noted in the historical section of the report. Also included in the case history might be test scores from other professionals who have evaluated the client previously. Some of these, such as IQ scores, are noted in the case history and constitute very sensitive information. If a client is being seen by another professional (e.g., psychologist, physician), this is outlined in the case history. The diagnostic report also includes all of the test results of the SLP evaluation including standard scores and percentile ranks of performance on various assessment instruments. Finally, the report will include the evaluator's interpretation of the test results and the formal diagnosis of a disorder. This report may also include recommendations for referrals to other professionals in addition to a diagnosis and prognosis. It is easy to see that no one would want such personal information to be compromised. Our clients assume that any information they divulge will be treated with confidentiality, and a professional should treat this obligation very seriously.

Rainy Day Reporting

Susan Pierce arrived at the university speech and hearing clinic parking lot just in time to grab the last parking space available. It was a rainy Monday morning and she was not looking forward to her back-to-back schedule of supervisory conferences with speech pathology practicum students. Susan had been a clinical supervisor for 5 years and thought she had "seen it all" with regard to student problems. Struggling to open her umbrella and exit her car at the same time, she immediately stepped into a large puddle adjacent to the driver's side door. It was then that she noticed the paper that was pinned squarely in the water beneath her fashionable black high-heeled pump. Through the water she read the smudged yet legible clinic letterhead; and under that was the section called "Identifying Information," which contained the client's name, address, telephone, and other personal information. Further down was a section devoted to case history, which described the devastation in the wake of a major stroke and the effects on the client's job and family. Although the type was a bit smeared, it was easy to read all the sensitive personal information that had been given in confidence to a caring clinician. Literally hundreds of people pass through this parking lot in a day, and Susan could only speculate how many of them might have paused to read this lost report. As you might anticipate, every report is signed by the student clinician and supervisor, and Susan's heart sank as she observed her own name at the bottom of the second page. This grim scenario probably began as an innocent lapse in safeguarding confidential information with a partially zipped backpack, unsnapped notebook, or papers being blown unobserved from the front seat of a vehicle. But innocent or not, such lapses in safeguarding information have repercussions and consequences. The chain of events can affect the client, the supervisor, the reputation of the clinic, and the perception of the student. Susan strode into the building, her lips drawn back into a thin red line, hoping she would see the student clinician responsible for this unforgivable breakdown in protecting client confidentiality.

Information on Diskettes and Flash Drives Used by Students

Many students maintain information about their client(s) on diskettes in order to keep track of the information more efficiently. Students should be very cautious about using these disks in computers outside of the university clinic or their own personal computers and should return the disks to the university clinic following the completion of their sessions with the client. Many students use flash drives that plug into the USB ports of computers. It is not uncommon for a student to have his "whole life" on that one flash drive, such as personal correspondence, classroom work, term papers, and drafts of clinical reports as well. The reason manufacturers put lanyards on those flash drives is that they are likely to be lost or misplaced because of their compact size. If you lose your flash drive you are not only losing your whole life but the lives of any clients who are mentioned in those files. If you keep any electronic copies of your reports, make sure they are in a safe place; even better, delete those files after the information is no longer of use.

The Hard Lesson of the Hard Drive

Candace Newman was a master of using time between classes to do her homework. If she had a free hour, she would go to one of the 10 student computer labs located across the large university campus. It was a great opportunity to work on term papers for core classes in English, history, sociology, and science. It was also a chance to work on clinical reports for several clients she was seeing in practicum at the university speech and hearing clinic. Candace had diagnostic reports and midterm treatment reports that were due to be turned in to her supervisor within a week. With only 5 minutes remaining before her next class, Candace hurriedly saved her document. She had done so much work on the report that she decided to check her personal computer disk to see if the document had actually been saved. When she looked at the directory for her disk, the report was not there. So she saved the report again and confirmed that it was, in

fact, on her disk. Unknown to Candace, however, her first attempt at saving the report ended up on the public computer's hard drive. Now the report, which detailed the history and personal information of Joey Dean, a child with fragile X syndrome, was available in a public computer lab for anyone to access. Maybe no one would pull the document up at all and the information would be lost in the maw of files on the hard drive. On the other hand, maybe someone would be curious about the file and access it to see what it was. Either way, Candace has planted a confidentiality time bomb that might come back to haunt her, the university clinic, her supervisor, and worst of all, Joey's family. Only time will tell.

Electronic Transmissions

Much of the communication between the university clinic and outside referral sources, allied health professionals, students and instructors, and even clients may be communicated via electronic mail (e-mail). Clinic personnel, as well as student clinicians, should be aware that this information may be read by someone other than the person or persons for whom it was intended. To this end, any and all attempts to protect our clients' privacy should be made. Identifying information such as file numbers or initials may be used instead of a client's name.

Authorization Forms

Most university clinics require clients to sign an authorization form, or "release" in order to evaluate and/or provide speech therapy services. This form is usually kept in the client's confidential file, and therefore is not subject to viewing by anyone other than clinic staff. At some university clinics that have a sliding fee schedule, prospective clients are required to report information on family size and personal income to qualify for reduced fees. Such financial information is obviously very sensitive and must be safeguarded.

Therapy Schedules

At our clinic, a comprehensive schedule of all client appointments is posted outside our front office so that anyone who needs to check the day and/or time of a therapy session can do so easily. Such a schedule should not contain client names, in that this information could be viewed by anyone entering the clinic. Instead, a file number may be used to identify each client. It is also important that students do not congregate and discuss clients in common areas.

Verbal Discussions

In a university setting it is not uncommon for students to communicate with one another in classes, before classes, while waiting for a client to arrive, or just walking down a corridor in the speech and hearing clinic. One of the things our students have in common is their experiences in classes and in clinical practicum. Thus, it may seem natural to discuss a client you are working with, especially if you are having a great deal of success or on the other hand if you are frustrated due to lack of progress. While you are having these conversations you never know who will be in a position to overhear what you say.

Foot in Mouth Disease

Toni and Trisha were standing by the restroom in the clinic hallway talking about one of their clients who had not had a very productive session.

"Man, he's a brat!" Trisha complained.

"Yeah, he was terrible today. I'm sure glad I don't have to take him home," Toni replied.

Trisha laughed as she sipped her Diet Coke. "And can you believe his mother thinks there's nothing wrong with him? What's up with that?"

About that time, the mother walks out of the restroom and into the hall where the students are standing. Trisha almost chokes on her Diet Coke, as Toni, red faced, picks up her cell phone and begins a text message to her boyfriend. Mom turns and walks down the hall, obviously hurt by their rude remarks. The students look at each other in disbelief. "Man, we really messed up that time," Toni mumbles.

The next week, the mother calls the clinic and cancels her son's therapy appointment. Then, she cancels the next one, and the next one, until it's almost mid-semester. Finally, when the clinical supervisor calls to ask her if there's a problem, she says, "Yes there certainly is, your students were saying terrible things about me and my son and I don't appreciate it one bit. I'll never come back to that clinic!"

Students should also be aware that danger of being overheard lurks outside the clinic environment as well. When you are at the mall, at a restaurant, in a nightclub, or at church you might be tempted to discuss your clinical work with a friend. If you use identifying information in these conversations there is always a chance that your client's friend, neighbor, coworker, teacher, or relative might just be at the adjacent table or strolling behind you in the mall. This is especially dangerous in small communities where people tend to know everything that is going on. *Thus, a good rule of thumb is if you have any doubt about whether to discuss information about a client, then don't!*

In this part of the chapter, we have been discussing confidentiality as it applies to the university clinic. The next sections will discuss the issue of confidentiality as it relates to medical and school settings.

MEDICAL SETTINGS

There are a number of medical settings in which speech/language evaluation and treatment take place: hospitals, long-term care facilities, skilled nursing facilities, and rehabilitation hospitals, to name a few. In our field, the term *medical setting* is generally used to refer to institutions that treat patients who have been diagnosed with any type of illness, injury, disease, or other condition that affects their speech, language, or swallowing function. These facilities are normally staffed by medical personnel such as doctors, nurses, therapists, and various other specialists. In general, a university clinic, public school, or private practice is not considered a medical setting due to the absence of any medically trained personnel.

However, there are exceptions, in that some university clinics are associated with teaching hospitals and therefore may consult with physicians or other medical professionals.

Most of the paperwork that contains client information in a medical setting is similar to paperwork seen in the university clinic (i.e., evaluation reports, therapy plans, progress notes, SOAP notes). In the university setting or private practice, each patient has a file or chart that is typically kept in the clinic office and the only professional who contributes to the chart is the SLP or audiologist. In medical facilities, the patient's chart is kept in a controlled central location so that the many different professionals involved in the patient's care can have access to it. Therefore, it is paramount that this information is kept confidential. It is also not a good idea to discuss a patient with anyone other than those involved in his care. Often, a patient in a medical setting is noncommunicative and is therefore at the mercy of a caregiver or facility staff to protect his privacy. In this case, the student clinician should be aware of the responsibility to protect the rights of the patient. Any violation of these rights is a direct violation of HIPAA and may result in fines and or imprisonment. Being regulated by HIPAA means that you must always be conscious of the *who, what, where,* and *when*: know *who* you can talk to, *what* you can talk about, *where* you can talk about it, and *when* it is appropriate to talk about it.

John Jacobs was a distinguished attorney who had a stroke in the middle of a trial while defending his client for a murder he did not commit. Right in the middle of his introductory remarks he slumped over the table and the bailiff called 911. As a result of his stroke, Mr. Jacobs could not talk at all but could think as clearly as ever. He was incontinent and forced to wear a hospital gown that was open in the back. People he did not know wandered in and out of his room with various missions involving respiration, speech, meals, and changing IVs. He was poked and prodded by everyone from social workers to student nurses. He had a roommate who continually turned the shared television up so loud that there was no time for personal reflection. So, here was John Jacobs, attorney–at–law, who had lost every last vestige of his personal privacy. But there was one more indignity to suffer. He began to cry as he listened to a conversation between two nursing students there to change his catheter. They talked about his personal history, his son who never visited, and even the client accused of murder who was ultimately convicted.

SCHOOL SETTINGS

The paperwork in the public schools differs significantly from the medical setting, university clinic, or private practice. This is due, in part, to the nature of the delivery of services, as well as to the federal laws that govern public schools and how they serve students with disabilities.

The Education of all Handicapped Children Act (EHA), also known as Public Law or PL-94-142, passed in 1975, mandated that all handicapped children between the ages of 3 and 21 receive a free, public education appropriate to their need, and in the least restrictive environment. In 1990, as part of its reauthorization by Congress, this law was renamed the Individuals with Disabilities Education Act or IDEA (PL 101-476). To that end, any child with a diagnosed communication disorder is covered under IDEA and entitled to free and appropriate individualized services (Haynes, Moran, & Pindzola, 2006).

Before a child can receive any special education services, including speech-language therapy, an extensive evaluation procedure is required. Once this evaluation process is complete, and it is determined that the child is eligible for special education services, an *individualized education plan* (IEP) must be written to meet the needs of the child. Any child with a communication disorder, who is receiving speech therapy services, will have an IEP. The IEP is unique to the school setting and is the cornerstone of a quality education for each child with a disability. (U.S. Department of Education, 2005)

In most school settings, the original copy of the IEP is kept in the student's confidential file in an administrative office. Copies of the IEP are usually kept by each teacher or professional who serves the student in the special education capacity, to ensure that all of the student's goals are being addressed.

Parents may, at any time, request a copy of the IEP, at which time the school must provide such. The parent may also request that the school release a copy of the IEP to other professionals who are working with the child, such as a university speech clinic. This is the case with many of our clients, as they are receiving services from their schools as well as at our clinic. As a speech pathology practicum student in the public schools, you will be expected to implement the goals outlined for each student with whom you are assigned to work. The school SLP will usually provide a copy of the student's IEP for you to follow. For more information, go to the the National Dissemination Center for Children and Youth with Disabilities (NICHCY) Web site (http://www.nichcy.org) for a detailed description of the law.

What is important to know regarding ethics and confidentiality is that any failure to implement the goals outlined in the student's IEP is a violation of federal law; therefore, each person who works with a student who has an IEP is accountable for the goals outlined therein, and this information is kept in a confidential space within the school building. Copies of a student's IEP should not be found floating around the school, or even worse, leaving the building!

Public school SLPs also keep many records in addition to the IEP. Each child will have a folder that includes various test results, treatment progress reports, weekly notes, and other forms of confidential information such as audio/video recordings. This information must be safeguarded as in any other setting until it is disposed of using appropriate methods.

We have tried to illustrate in the present chapter that there is an intimate relationship between professional ethics, protecting confidentiality, and professional communication. These relationships cross work settings and are *always* an important factor in the daily conduct of clinical work. Thus, as a student moving from one setting to another you will always carry with you a concern about patient privacy and confidentiality. It is not a question of whether confidentiality will be a major issue, because it always is. One of your first concerns in a new practicum setting is to find out how the facility handles client privacy issues and make sure you religiously adhere to those procedures.

SECTION II

Professional Written Communication

4 Diagnostic Reports

This section begins our discussion of professional written communication in speech-language pathology. What is important to know is that the diagnostic report is sometimes the first communication someone reads about a client or patient, and therefore, it must be concise yet detailed and relevant to the patient's disorder. We have had students tell us that the format we like for them to use is different from that of our other colleagues who are faculty in the same training program. Miller and Groher (1990) state that the best type of report "will paint a verbal picture of a clinical case and lead the reader or listener through the collection of pertinent data to a logical diagnostic conclusion" (p. 243).

If there is one concept that is important to both professional written communication and professional verbal communication it is *organization*. Without organization, one cannot write a coherent report, plan treatment goals/objectives, participate effectively in a multidisciplinary staffing, interview a parent, provide evaluation results, or counsel clients. Organization is one of the major variables that distinguishes professional from nonprofessional communication. Thus, successful beginning students as well as veteran clinicians have one thing in common: They think a lot before they write or talk.

As indicated in the title, this chapter is concerned with diagnostic report writing, and this type of report is an excellent example of why a good clinician needs to be organized. Think for a moment what happens in a diagnostic evaluation. Haynes and Pindzola (2008) illustrate that a variety of information is gathered in an evaluation. For example, you may have accumulated data in the following areas: (a) case history information, (b) prior tests and reports, (c) observation of client behavior, (d) interview findings, (e) nonstandardized testing, and (f) standardized testing. In some of these areas such as standardized testing, there may have been administration of multiple instruments. Thus, an evaluation gathers multiple sources of information, and the good diagnostician must take these disparate sources of data and synthesize them to arrive at a diagnosis. In some cases the six sources of information may disagree. For instance, a child may pass a standardized language test but exhibit many errors in a spontaneous speech sample (nonstandardized testing.) The evaluator must reconcile all of these types of information to arrive at a diagnosis. Imagine if you will a desk containing case history forms, notes from a parent interview, transcripts of a communication sample, prior reports from other professionals, multiple test forms, and notes from a behavioral observation, and you will see how important organization is to approaching a diagnostic report. So far, we have only mentioned the types of data you have gathered in an assessment. The diagnostic report must not only summarize all of the types of data that have been gathered, but the clinician must arrive at a diagnosis, prognosis, suggestions for further testing, clinical management suggestions, and a rationale for referral to other professionals if appropriate. Again, as the available information is surveyed, the competent clinician is thinking about the pieces that can be used to address areas such as prognosis, treatment suggestions, and justification for referral. This requires approaching the task with an organizational structure in mind. In addition to organization, appropriate terminology is key to writing a professional diagnostic report. We will be illustrating some important concepts related to organization, format, and language used in diagnostic reports in the following pages. This is not meant to be a workbook for students to use in developing report writing style. We will also not take a disorder-specific approach to reporting and provide examples from the many different disorder areas in the field. There are many fine sources that do a competent job of providing practice in these areas (Meyer, 2004; Pannbacker, Middleton, Vekovius, & Sanders, 2001). Our intention is to talk about the variables involved in diagnostic reporting and provide some limited examples. It is important to remember that no matter how many examples are provided in a textbook, the setting in which you are working will probably do things a bit differently than the illustrations. We think that the formats, organization process, and language are the primary determinants of professional written communication and those are what we will discuss here. We also believe that it is important to illustrate diagnostic reporting as it exists across work settings at the university, medical facility, and school system.

THE ORGANIZATIONAL FRAMEWORK OF A DIAGNOSTIC REPORT

Since we have indicated that organization is so important to professional written communication, we will discuss issues of format first. Not only is format important to organizing the writing of a report, it is also helpful in assembling all the information you have gathered during an evaluation. You can think of the sections of a report as boxes or bins in which you can place information you will later write about. One caveat before we begin: While there is always certain information that is "required" in a diagnostic report, various clinics may subdivide these evaluation summaries differently in terms of headings. There are many ways to slice and dice the information in a diagnostic report, and we will be presenting our own unique format in this text; keep in mind that we are providing an organizational framework to act as a general guide. Just remember that you will be using different headings depending on where you are working, but the information we mention will all be included somewhere in the report. Let's look at the typical sections in a diagnostic report:

■ **Identifying Information:** This is basic demographic information such as name, age, date of birth, case/file number, gender, address, date of the evaluation, and telephone number. It is obviously important to identify the client completely as well as when the evaluation was performed.

■ **Background Information:** This includes case history information from forms, prior test results, reports from other professionals, and notes from interviewing the client, family members, or parents. The importance and type of historical information varies considerably based on the type of disorder that is present and the age of the client. For instance, neonatal, birth, and developmental history is more important for a 2-year-old than for an older child or adult. The vocational history is more important for an adult who has had a stroke than for a teenager who is still in school. Medical background is more important for clients with a medically-based disorder than those with more behaviorally-based problems. The clinician must look at all of the case history data and interview protocols and determine which information is the most relevant to the focus of the evaluation. This section of the diagnostic report also includes the principal reason the person was referred for the evaluation. Embedded somewhere in the background information should be a statement of why the client came for services. While this statement is not a separate section of the report, it is important to mention the client's perspective in the background information. Utilizing the "statement of the problem" will help to focus the assessment on the topic of primary concern and will determine test selection for the evaluation.

■ **Biological Bases of Communication:** What we refer to in this section is auditory acuity, structure/function of the oral mechanism, and a cursory examination of neurological integrity. Most evaluations include a hearing screening to rule out auditory acuity problems or to justify referral to an audiologist for a full evaluation. A statement of the results of the audiological screening goes in this section and usually provides information on the frequencies screened and the attenuation level of the audiometer. Especially in cases where motoric or structural abnormalities are suspected, we perform an oral-peripheral examination, which tests the structure and function of the oral mechanism. We also note any possible neurological symptoms such as paralysis, weakness, drooling, deficits in fine and gross motor skill, or client reports of seizures or head injury. This section can be quite brief if there are no remarkable findings. Obviously, the more abnormalities that are noted in structure or function of the speech mechanism, the longer this section will become.

- **Basic Communication Processes of Language, Articulation, Voice/Resonance, and Fluency that Are within Normal Limits:** When a person undergoes an evaluation for a possible communication disorder, it is assumed that the diagnostician has examined *all basic processes of communication*. For instance, we do not know that a client referred for an articulation problem does not have a language disorder as well. Thus, it is imperative that at some point in the evaluation the clinician take the time to assess, if only informally, the four areas of language, articulation, voice/resonance, and fluency. In most cases we will not administer formal tests in the four basic areas because we can see from nonstandardized tasks such as conversation that there are no significant problems. For example, a child referred for misarticulations can be seen to have normal vocal production and fluency from listening to a conversational sample for voice quality and dysfluencies. Especially in the university practicum setting, students might be asked to administer tests in several of the basic communication processes for the purpose of gaining experience in test administration. However, in other settings, formal testing of all areas of communication is often omitted and not reported on because they are not areas of major concern. In those cases, a clinician might not test articulation in a case that was referred for fluency, especially if no misarticulations were noted in

spontaneous conversation. The bottom line here is that the diagnostic report must address, however briefly, the basic areas of communication to show that we have considered each of these as an area of possible communication disorder. This could be a brief statement such as, "No abnormalities were noted in the client's voice production, resonance, articulation, or fluency."

- **Diagnostic Test Results Focusing on the Area(s) of Concern:** The bulk of the diagnostic report will involve detailing the test results on the patient's area of major concern. If that concern is a child language disorder, we will be reporting the results of many standardized tests and the results of different analyses of a language sample (e.g., mean length of utterance, type-token ratio, syntactic complexity, grammatical errors, pragmatic difficulties). If the concern is a fluency disorder, we will be administering and reporting many measurements of overt behaviors (e.g., frequency and type of dysfluency) and indicators of covert dimensions related to stuttering (such as feelings, attitudes, avoidances). A person whose primary concern is hoarseness will be administered many behavioral and instrumental measures of phonation during a variety of tasks ranging from prolonging vowels to connected speech. It only makes sense that the diagnostic report will devote the most space and focus to the topic of major concern.

- **Clinical Impressions:** In this section of a report, the clinician interprets the different test results and background information to arrive at a diagnosis and prognosis. The section is longer when there is disagreement among the different types of clinical data because the clinician has to explain why certain results are at odds.

- **Summary and Recommendations:** This section is the most frequently read portion of a diagnostic report, especially by busy professionals. The evaluation is briefly summarized and specific recommendations for treatment, no treatment, or referral are detailed.

The organization of a diagnostic report, whether written for an adult or child client, will usually contain information from the sections presented above.

While an evaluation done in any work setting is concerned with the same basic information we have just described, diagnostic reporting across work settings is not exactly the same. The principal difference revolves around the length of the reports. Reports in medical and school settings tend to be shorter due to (a) limitations in the use of narrative explanations and (b) report forms that limit length due to use of check boxes to indicate the presence/absence of abnormality, or a limited space allocated to note test scores. We will be discussing these versions of diagnostic reports in later sections.

UNIVERSITY CLINIC

Length, Content, and Format

As you probably know by now, the university clinic requires students to write detailed reports summarizing the evaluation process. In the university setting, most students begin by learning to write long narrative reports that in some cases may be five or more pages in length, depending on the type of case. One reason these reports are longer than in other settings is that students are often asked to administer tests that are not particularly necessary for diagnosis but are selected to give the student experience with testing. A second reason these reports are long is that students need to gain experience with professional writing. At some point in your career you might be asked to write a detailed report as part of a legal proceeding or to explain a very complicated case to another professional to whom a client is referred. In these instances, knowing how to provide clinical detail in a professional manner is important. Another reason for longer reports is that most university clinics perform comprehensive speech and language evaluations, sometimes lasting up to 2 hours. Some other settings may have evaluation time slots that extend only 20 to 30 minutes. You can simply get more testing done in 2 hours, and then you have to report the results. A final reason for the longer reports is that in the training setting, we can ask students to do more time-intensive tasks such as transcribing language samples and analyzing video recordings of play behaviors. These are important skills for students to

develop. Even though such analyses represent the highest level of validity and expertise in our field, they may not be done in medical or school settings. In general, a person in a private practice, school system, or medical facility may not have the time to perform such an in-depth evaluation. However, because the university clinic is a training facility, students may be exposed to the full gamut of evaluation procedures. Thus, in the university training program you will be writing the longest of your clinical reports and you will need to learn how to pare them down in other settings. It is better, however, to know the long version before you move into more abbreviated clinical writing. As Shipley and McAfee (1998) point out, the consolation for you, the student, is that once you graduate and practice professionally, you will be able to pick and choose aspects you like from all the different models and develop your own unique style of writing.

Now we will address the content of the report in a university setting. We gather so much information in a diagnostic evaluation that it is sometimes difficult to determine what is important and what is not. So, what are the ingredients of a good report? How do you get to a logical diagnostic conclusion? Let's start with first things first. A thorough description of the patient's case history is imperative. I want to learn as much as I can about this person in the first paragraph of this report. Just as if I was reading a good book, I want something to draw me in, keep me interested, and be informative. Rambling, unimportant information is not going to keep my attention, but concise, detailed, relevant information will. Identifying information such as name, address, telephone number, and date of birth are required and it is critical to insure this information is correct. Sections such as background information and statement of the problem are not always straightforward and the clinician will have to make some judgment calls on certain issues. For instance, is it more important that Jimmy likes to play soccer, or that he "can't remember anything" since he fell and hit his head on the driveway? We would vote for the head injury. It is always good to preserve the patient's or parent's statement of the problem. This is the statement that helps to guide the evaluation toward the topic of immediate concern. So, if you ask a parent why she brought her son in for an evaluation, she might say,

"John has been struggling with saying his words. It's like he gets stuck and you can see the frustration on his face. I'm worried that he is beginning to stutter." That is the kind of quote that belongs in a diagnostic report because it helps to focus the evaluation and justify all of the tests and tasks you performed to assess fluency under various conditions. Speech pathology practicum students often make the mistake of not including enough pertinent information or, on the other hand, adding information that is unnecessary. A good rule of thumb is to report any information that you feel could impact speech, language, or swallowing function and describe it so that it makes sense.

Regarding other data to be mentioned in a diagnostic report, clearly the format sections we mentioned earlier will dictate the inclusion of certain types of information. Obviously, test results from standardized and nonstandardized information are important to include. After reporting test results, the diagnostic report should relate clinical impressions, summarize the findings, and make recommendations or referrals. Usually the reporting of scores or behavioral data involves listing numerical information and perhaps some behavioral description. Clinical impressions and recommendations tend to be more narrative in nature but still based firmly on the historical information, test results, and behavioral observation.

Writing Style

In this section we will get down to the nuts and bolts of professional written communication and discuss terminology and common errors students commit in clinical reports.

> *Student 1:* "I hate writing reports because my supervisor always changes everything I write."
>
> *Student 2:* "Yeah, I know what you mean. Mine looks like it's bleeding to death when I get it back from my supervisor—red everywhere!"
>
> *Student 1:* "She never likes the way I say things. It's like she thinks I'm stupid or something."

Has this scenario happened to you? More than likely, if you are a student in a university SLP program, it has. What is it about reports that makes them so difficult? Why is it that certain things have to be said a "certain way" or they are wrong? The truth of the matter is, what is written by students is not always wrong; it is just that reports are different when written by different people and across work settings. The format, style, length, and degree of detail needed for a diagnostic report varies across settings, university programs, and sometimes even supervisors in the same setting (Shipley & McAfee, 1998).

Some 30 years ago we wrote an article entitled, "The Agony of Report Writing: A New Look at an Old Problem" (Haynes & Hartman, 1975). Interestingly, this article is still quoted extensively in the most recent textbooks dealing with professional writing (Moon, 2004; Pannbacker et al., 2001). The reason that the article remains relevant is not that it was particularly groundbreaking or prescient, but because clinical writing still inflicts a good deal of pain on students in training, just as it always has. In that article we outlined two areas that still have the imprint of clinical relevance to students. One area was a professional terminology generator that provided examples of the kinds of terms used in clinical reports. There is a certain type of language used in professional communication and there is no reason to keep it a secret from our students. In the present text (see Appendix A), we have further developed our terminology generator to include general terms from specific disorder areas, and we have expanded the general terminology section to include updated terms. Students can use the professional terminology generator in several ways. First, when you are searching for a term to use in writing a report and you cannot think of one, you can look at the items in Appendix A for possible examples to use. Second, you can use the generator to reduce redundancy in reports. For example, there is redundancy in the following: "The client was not stimulable for any error phonemes. The client responded well to phonetic placement of bilabial stop consonants." Choosing another term to refer to the client would reduce redundancy in the two sentences ("The client was not stimulable for any error phonemes; however, he responded well to phonetic placement of bilabial stop consonants."). There are many ways to say that a patient "has" a particular condition (e.g., *shows, exhibits, manifests, demonstrates, displays*, etc.) and you do not have to redundantly use the same term in every sentence.

There are also "professional tone words" in the generator that are often the variable that separates professional clinical communication from everyday speech. We encourage you to incorporate professional terminology in your reports from the beginning and not rely on your clinical supervisor to change what you have written to increase its professional tone.

Common Errors

Many sources discuss common mistakes that students make in their early report writing (Haynes & Hartman, 1975; Haynes & Pindzola, 2008; Knepflar, 1978; Meitus, 1983; Moore, 1969; Shipley & McAfee, 1998). We feel that these frequent errors should not be kept a secret from students, but should be mentioned so that they can be proactive in clinical writing. Some of the following are errors mentioned in the above references:

1. **Redundancy:** This refers to the use of the same terms within a sentence and across abutting sentences. Redundancy can also refer to repetition of the same concept or idea. For example, the following sentences basically say the same thing: *The results of this evaluation suggest that Joey will have little difficulty in correcting his articulation problem. Joey's prognosis is good.*

2. **Wordiness:** Every attempt should be made to state diagnostic information in the most economical way possible. Reports are no place for wordy descriptions. This is why we use professional terminology. Instead of saying, "The client could not produce the phonemes that were in error even with multiple trials of maximum multisensory stimulation and modeling," it is enough to say, "The client was not stimulable for any errored phonemes."

3. **Lack of Professional Terminology:** As we illustrate in the terminology generator in Appendix A there are certain professional terms that are typically used in reports. As we stated earlier, a common error is to refer to phonemes as "sounds."

4. **Lack of Objectivity and Not Separating Fact from Opinion:** Reports should include objective information and not unsubstantiated assumptions on the part of the clinician. Reasonable interpretation of test scores is fairly objective in terms of characterizing a client's performance in relation to standard scores. A person who scores 2 standard deviations below the mean could easily be considered to exhibit a disorder in the area tested. If we are talking about parent reports, we should couch these with phrases such as "the parent reported . . . the mother stated." If we are talking about our own opinions, this should be stated as such ("It is the opinion of the examiner that Mary is not highly motivated for treatment."). This should be followed by a description of behaviors that support the clinician's observation such as the client's reluctance to enter the treatment room, crying when entering the clinical setting, and screaming, "I hate coming here," at the beginning of every session.

5. **Lack of Organization and Sequence:** Make sure that the appropriate information is included in the correct section of your report. For example, do not bring up history information in the clinical impressions section. A report should be organized in such a way that it flows from background information to test results to clinical impressions and finally to recommendations.

6. **Ambiguity:** A sentence such as, "The client did not perform well on the motor speech tasks," does not really tell us anything specific about performance. The client may not have tried very hard on the task or might have shown serious motoric deficits. It would be better to specify how many syllables were produced in 10 seconds.

7. **Tense Errors:** Typically, the case history portion of the report is written in past tense. Later, when discussing clinical impressions and recommendations, you can switch to more active sentence constructions since you are talking about the present and future.

8. **Spelling and Typographical Errors:** In this age of spell-checkers and grammatical screeners in word processing programs, there is no excuse for spelling and typographical errors in clinical reports. Submitting a report with these types of errors reflects poorly on the professionalism of the clinician. If we cannot trust your spelling and grammar, how much credibility can we

assign to your reporting of test scores and historical information?

9. **Wrong Use of Abbreviations:** While it is acceptable to use an abbreviation in a report, it should always be initially defined the first time it is used. A child might be administered the Goldman-Fristoe Test of Articulation (GFTA-2). If it is defined, as in the previous sentence, then it is all right to use GFTA-2 in later portions of the report.

10. **Use of Contractions and Informal Language:** Reports are no place to use contracted forms (e.g., *can't, won't, we'll, he'll,* etc.). Most authorities recommend using the fully formed versions of words that are amenable to contraction. Also, the use of informal, shortened versions of words such as "rehab" for rehabilitation is typically not recommended. Obviously, slang terminology is not acceptable in reports.

Do Not Forget Your Audience

Clinical reports end up in the hands of many different types of people. It is not possible to write a report that will be equally understood by your colleagues in SLP and a parent with limited educational experience. Another professional (e.g., psychologist, classroom teacher) may not understand terms that are unique to communication disorders, but if they are truly professional they will have encountered our terms before or will look them up. Certainly, when we receive reports from psychologists, they do not hesitate to use terminology unique to psychology. One solution would be to write the report to the lowest common denominator of audiences and remove all professional terms. This would help laypeople understand the report, but it would marginalize our profession. We have worked for many years to raise our profession to the same standard as other health-related professions, and part of that involves our style of reporting. One does not see psychologists, educational evaluation specialists, physical therapists, physicians, and occupational therapists write reports without professional language. If that were the case, a psychologist would have to explain IQ and testing methods in the report so that it would be understandable to laypersons. There are, however, schools

of thought in report writing that suggest we should generate reports that are "parent-friendly" or "family-friendly," omitting professional terms or including definitions and explanations of concepts referred to in the report. In some ways this is good for the family, but it makes our profession seem less than it is. A family-friendly report certainly would not represent our profession as well if sent to a psychologist or physician. Discipline-specific terms exist because they allow us to refer to phenomena in an efficient and professional way. Thus, it is important for you to remember where the report is going to be sent and who is primarily going to profit from reading it. If it is going in the university clinic file, it should be written professionally for another SLP. If it is going to a public school SLP, again, it should be written professionally. If the report is going to a professional from another discipline you should consider this while writing and define terms you feel may be unique. In medical or school settings, however, most people who work there share common terminology and freely use medical or educational terms because they communicate most efficiently. One compromise is that some clinics write reports for the clinical file and then write a separate letter to parents summarizing the results of the evaluation in less technical terms. There is no one way to write reports that has been agreed upon by clinics and work settings throughout the country. So, our best advice is to consider your primary audience and be as professional as possible. In some cases it may mean drafting several versions of your findings for various audiences either in the form of alternate reports or summary letters for parents. Ultimately, there must be a balance between communicating information and communicating professionally. One thing is for certain: You should not buy *The Big Book of Vocabulary* and learn words such as *magnanimous* or *obfuscation* and then amaze your colleagues by placing them in a clinical report. According to Haynes and Pindzola (2008), "A diagnostic report is no place to display your learning or to parade a large vocabulary. Pedantic reports are misunderstood or unread (p. 377)."

In Appendices B and C we provide examples of each section of a diagnostic report, based on the evaluation of a child and an adult. Through your graduate training, you will be exposed to various types of assessment based on specific disorders; therefore, we will not provide examples of a diagnostic report for every disorder in this text. In the next sections we will expand our discussion of diagnostic reporting to other settings beyond the university.

MEDICAL SETTING

A diagnostic report in a hospital, nursing home, or rehabilitation facility will most likely look very different from a report in the university clinic. The most noticeable differences will be the amount of information included and the format. Most medical facilities use a one-page report, and some even use a fill in the blank or checklist format, in which the SLP simply marks the areas that are appropriate for each patient. We have included several examples of diagnostic reporting forms from a medical setting in Appendices D through F.

Most students who complete a practicum in a medical setting are initially thrilled when they see how "easy" these diagnostic forms are to fill out. The only drawback is you have to know exactly what information is relevant before you can accurately complete the form—this is where your practice in writing lengthy diagnostic reports comes in handy. You have already practiced figuring out what information is most pertinent and reporting it in a narrative format; now, you can apply that information to the new format. It's easy, right? Not so fast. Many of the supervisors in the medical setting that we talked to while researching the present textbook told us that students still have difficulty "filling out the form." What we learned is that students are still tentative about which boxes to check or that they are not very familiar with the medical terminology. To help you in this area, we will provide a list of the most commonly used medical terms and symbols in Appendix J.

While knowledge of terminology will be of some assistance to beginning students, familiarity with terms alone will not alleviate your tentativeness as your pen or mouse hovers over a series of check boxes. Your greatest ally will be a logical organization of your case history data and assessment data and clear thinking about the results of the evaluation. The same procedures you went through in the university clinic are important to use in understanding the case, no matter how brief the report format. If you must choose between *aphasia* and *motor speech disorder*, you still must have thought through the evidence from your evaluation before checking the appropriate box. The important thing is that you understand *why* you are checking a particular box on a diagnostic form.

In most cases, a diagnostic report in a hospital, nursing home, or rehabilitation facility will include the same basic information (give or take a few sections) as a diagnostic report you would write in a university clinic. These days, however, most of what you "report" in one of these settings will involve checking boxes, filling in the blanks, or writing a short description on a computer generated form. Or, if you are at a more technologically advanced facility, you will sit down at a computer, open a software program, and point and click your way to describing your patient's speech, language or swallowing problem. You then click "print" and your diagnostic report is ready!

Do not get too far ahead of yourself, though. It is still very important that you have adequate knowledge of what is important in order to be a good diagnostic reporter. As long as you use the information provided thus far, you should be on the right track.

PUBLIC SCHOOL SETTING

Reports in the public schools vary greatly from the typical report that you would see in a medical setting, private practice, or university clinic. The information gleaned from a diagnostic evaluation may not be written down in a standard diagnostic format, as has been discussed in the previous sections, although we have seen this done in certain states. We have found that in many school systems, once the evaluation is completed, the information is compiled, discussed by the IEP team, and then transferred to an eligibility form. What you as a practicum student in the schools will see is this eligibility form. The form will include all areas of assessment, dates and names of the assessments, as well as the results. In addition, the student's strengths and needs will be included.

An example of an eligibility form is included in Appendix G. According to school personnel, determining strengths and needs is one of the most difficult tasks for speech pathology practicum students. Thus, the challenge of diagnostic reports in the schools is not so much in reporting the test findings, but in determining the needs of each child, based on a comprehensive evaluation.

Let's talk about what this comprehensive evaluation entails. In most public school systems, you are required to administer at least two formal assessments in language and one formal assessment in speech. The language scores will then be calculated, and, based on the standard score, it will be determined if a child is eligible for services. Eligibility determination differs by state and in some cases even by school system within the same state. Typically, a language or articulation standard score must be more than 1.5 to 2 standard deviations (SD) below the mean in order for a child to qualify for services in either speech or language disorders. Most school systems require the SLP to administer a comprehensive language assessment, one that tests both receptive and expressive language. Then, if a child shows a deficit in expressive language, for instance, the SLP must administer a formal assessment that specifically targets expressive language. According to IDEA, informal assessments can also be made part of the evaluation process. This is especially important in cases where a student may pass standardized tests but evidence errors in a spontaneous speech sample. Although informal assessments may not be considered by some school systems when determining if a child has a language delay, obtaining a language sample can be an invaluable resource in helping to "nail down" even more specific areas of deficit in children who are language impaired. Parents also have the right to seek a second opinion from a source outside the school system if they disagree with the determination of eligibility or diagnosis of their child (Haynes, Moran, & Pindzola, 2006). Also, it is important to remember that there is a significant difference between arriving at a diagnosis and determining eligibility. Diagnosis involves using standardized and nonstandardized testing to determine the existence of a communication disorder and make specific recommendations for treatment. Eligibility determina-tion is largely an administrative operation that allows school systems to select with whom they will work. These two operations are quite different. One can have a communication disorder and may not qualify for services in the school system if it determines the disorder has no impact on educational progress or if test scores do not indicate enough of a deficit to meet criteria for eligibility.

Formal assessment is also important when evaluating a child with a fluency disorder in order to determine if the severity of the disorder warrants intervention; however, this assessment should not be limited to fluency counts, percentage of stuttered syllables, or other formal measures of severity alone. Assessment of stuttering should include discussion of the child's attitudes and emotions about her stuttering and consider the overall impact of the disorder on participation in her life (Yarrus, 2007).

Frequently, a child will be identified as having a voice problem during the course of a speech, language, or fluency evaluation. Because this is a subjective judgment by the speech-language clinician, it may be necessary to refer the child for medical follow-up with an ear, nose, and throat specialist (ENT). Often, the school clinician will initiate a vocal abuse awareness and/or vocal hygiene program that will be included in the child's speech goals.

Once the evaluations are finished, an eligibility form is completed. Each assessment that has been administered to the child (and the completion date) is listed, along with a description of the child's strengths and needs in each area. From there, goals are developed that target deficit areas (whether in speech, language, voice, or fluency) and benchmarks are established that will enable the SLP to help the child meet goals in the most timely and efficient manner. Figure 4–1 will give you a better idea of how the diagnostic process works in the public schools.

This chapter would not be complete without a mention of computerized report writing. As you can well imagine, there are software programs for generating almost any type of document that exists. This is also true for the field of speech-language pathology. Many hospitals, private practices, and school agencies now use computer programs to generate diagnostic reports, treatment reports (see Chapter 5), progress notes, and IEPs. There are many programs available

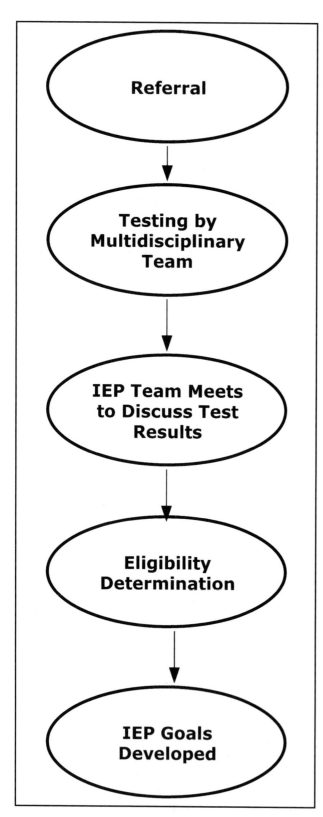

Figure 4–1. Diagnostic process in the public school setting.

in today's market, and sometimes knowing which one to choose can be challenging. Pannbacker et al. (2001, p. 69) remind us, "It is important when considering report writing software to evaluate the quality of reports as well as their applicability for each individual clinical circumstance." In the public schools, it has become commonplace for special educators, administrators, teachers, and SLPs to use IEP software. There are a myriad of programs available for generating IEPs, and depending on the state you are in, you may or may not be exposed to these. It is good to know about these programs and the ways that computer generated reports may increase the efficiency of documentation of service delivery. Several software programs for medical and school-based agencies are presented in the box below.

Report Writing Software

The Speech & Language Report Writer, by
    Clinician's Magician, Ltd.
P.O. Box 426
Bedford, NY 10506
http://www.cliniciansmagician.com

Wordweaver Report Writing Software
Data Morphosis
118 South Ridge St., Suite 196
Rye Brook, NY 10573
http://www.datamorphosis.com

IEP and Report Writer
Parrot Software
P.O. Box 250755
West Bloomfield, MI 48325-0755
http://www.parrotsoftware.com

Special Education Report Writing Software (eSped)
(Generates IEP forms)
800-365-0114
http://www.esped.com

QuickWriter
Ewing Solutions
4020 E. Weldon
Phoenix, AZ 85018
800-211-5882
https://www.quickwriter.com

It is important to remember, however, that *you* are still the clinician and the computer programs referred to above cannot think for you. This is especially critical in report writing programs that actually generate sentences based on information the clinician is prompted to provide. Always proofread the computer-generated report for accuracy and do not let the algorithms put words in your mouth, especially if they could be misinterpreted by those reading the report. No matter how a report is generated, it is always the responsibility of the clinician to insure clarity and accuracy.

In closing, what is most important for you, the practicum student, to realize is that thorough assessment of the patient or client, along with a clear description of the results and implications of that assessment, is the first step in providing the most efficacious plan of care. In order to function as a competent provider of services, you must begin with an accurate, professional, and meaningful description of your patient/client's needs.

5 Documenting Treatment Planning: Goals, Objectives, and Rationales

Speech-language pathology is an extremely diverse and ever-changing profession that encompasses a vast array of disorders and individuals from infants to geriatrics. Clinicians are beginning to specialize in the assessment and treatment of various disorders; so much so that certification in specific areas is becoming commonplace. At the same time, ongoing research, in the form of evidence-based practice (EBP), is opening doors to new avenues of treatment and new ways of understanding disorders of communication. Thus, the field of communication disorders is constantly changing. It may be daunting to you, a student, to imagine becoming competent in every area of this diverse field. However, it should be of some comfort to know that where there is change, there is also some consistency. What does *not* change is the fact that treatment of communication disorders must be planned, based on a thorough assessment, executed in a way that is efficacious and practical, and reported in a meaningful way. This chapter will focus on the process of establishing measurable goals and objectives and providing the rationales to back them up. We will focus on each of the various work settings and the way in which treatment planning is similar and different for each. We will also define a rationale and discuss why it is important to be able to explain why we make clinical decisions. The reason we have to address these issues in a textbook on professional communication is that you will be asked repeatedly to communicate goals and rationales verbally and in many types of reports, including treatment plans, progress summaries, and other forms as part of your clinical training.

In your coursework you have no doubt dealt with the concept that thought and mental organization underlie the language we use to communicate ideas. Thus, your verbal and written communication is organized by how you think about the topic of interest. We raised this issue in the previous chapter on diagnostic reports by saying that *organization* is key to developing professional clinical writing. In the case of treatment efforts, you must develop a principled way of thinking about goals and procedures before you can coherently talk or write about them. The process of thinking about a client's long-term goal provides you with an ultimate target that will be achieved when you dismiss the person from treatment. The short-term goals are the steps that you follow in a systematic way to approach the target. In psychology, this is known as successive (or progressive) approximation. We cannot expect that a client will achieve the long-term goal right away, but rather will move toward it in a systematic fashion. In fact, the whole concept of successive approximation is based on the notion that one cannot achieve long-term objectives without accomplishing short-term goals. They are the baby steps that allow a person to build competence on one level so that he can perform at higher levels. Clinicians must put a great deal of thought into identifying and sequencing goals of treatment so that they represent a hierarchy of difficulty leading to the ultimate long-term objective. If you have thought through the process, you will have a lot less difficulty writing a treatment plan or explaining what you are doing with a client to parents, family members, or observers of your treatment sessions. In the first part of this chapter, we will discuss goals and objectives and why they are an integral part of speech and language therapy reporting. We should note that our purpose in this chapter is not to provide examples of goal writing for every disorder that you might encounter in clinical practicum. Our mission here is to talk about the process of goal writing and how it drives your professional communication about the client.

Figure 5-1 shows the components involved in writing goals for a particular client. One component is your background knowledge gained from academic coursework. For example, you need information about normal development of the communication parameter that is affected in the client you are working with to determine the order in which normally-developing individuals acquire the skill. This can be a powerful indicator of the difficulty involved in skill acquisition, and normal development is often used as a guideline in ordering treatment goals. Another aspect of background knowledge is information about the particular disorder your client exhibits. For example, if it is phonology, you should know about the types of phonological errors commonly seen in children with disorders. You should also know about assessment and treatment procedures for use in dealing with phonological impairments. Thus, there is no substitute for background knowledge in writing goals because this information helps you to select treatment targets, sequence them in order of difficulty, and choose appropriate tasks to use in the conduct of therapy.

A second component in writing goals is specific knowledge of your client's current level of performance. This again emphasizes the importance of a thorough evaluation so that you will know exactly what the client can and cannot do with regard to phonological production, as in the previous example. The results of an evaluation may also impact your setting of long-term goals. For example, if a multidisciplinary evaluation revealed that your client has cognitive limitations such as mental retardation, a long-term goal of perfect intelligibility in complex sentences may not be realistic. The third component of writing goals is the basic process we will introduce on the following page in which we specify certain information as part of crafting observable, measurable be-

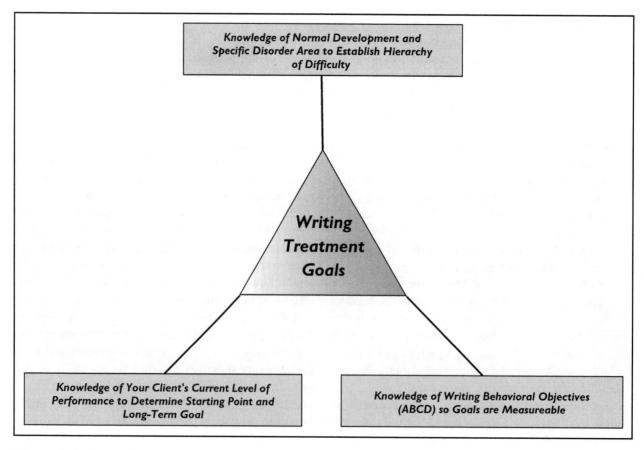

Figure 5–1. Prerequisite components of writing treatment goals.

havioral objectives. You should be able to see from Figure 5–1 that if any component is missing, the clinician will be at a loss to develop appropriate goals. It should also be apparent that a single chapter on writing goals cannot address all three components in Figure 5–1. We will focus only on the mechanics of writing behavioral objectives in this chapter and leave it to you to combine classroom information with these guidelines to arrive at measurable goals. We will also illustrate how these goals are similar and different in their appearance across practicum settings.

WHAT ARE LONG-TERM AND SHORT-TERM GOALS?

After an evaluation is completed, and before beginning a program of intervention, you will have to establish the goals that you will be working toward in therapy. The essence of intervention planning is the determination of long-term intervention goals and the development of procedures by which to achieve them. Klein and Moses (1994) define an intervention goal as "a potential achievement by an individual with a speech-language dysfunction directed toward the improvement of speech-language performance (p. 3)." The first step in planning treatment involves setting long-term goals, which will stipulate what you ultimately want your client to achieve. Once your long-term goals are established, you can then go on to the second step, which is to prioritize behaviors that will lead the client toward achievement of the long-term goals.

An example of a long-term goal is:

■ The client will produce all age-appropriate phonemes in spontaneous connected speech in order to improve speech intelligibility.

An example of a short-term goal is:

■ The client will spontaneously produce /t/ in the initial position of words while looking at picture cards with 90% accuracy in the clinical setting.

According to Klein and Moses (1994) a short-term goal is "a linguistic achievement that has been given priority within a hierarchy of achievements required for the realization of the long-term goal (p. 130)." In other words, the short-term goals are made up of *specific* behaviors you want to target in therapy that will enable your client to achieve long-term goals. The term *given priority* means that you have chosen these behaviors to be worked on first, assuming they will result in the most effective course of treatment. In the previous example, the short-term goal of "correct production of /t/ in words" is the first step in helping the client to produce age-appropriate phonemes that will improve overall intelligibility.

As the name implies, short-term refers to a definitive period of time. Obviously, we would not want to generate all of the possible steps leading from the client's current level of performance to the achievement of a long-term goal. That might entail scores of individual steps if you consider all of the different levels of language ranging from phoneme production to complex sentences, and all of the task levels from imitative to spontaneous conversation. Not only would this be unwieldy, but it would not take into account the possibility of generalization and spontaneous learning on the part of the client, which might make it possible to skip planned levels of training. Thus, we limit our short-term goals to a well-defined window of time. For example, the amount of time designated for achieving a short-term goal and the number of short-term goals are often determined by where the therapy is taking place. In the university clinic, the goal may be for a semester; in a hospital, it may be for a few days or a week; and in a long-term care facility, it may last until the patient's insurance stops paying for services. Generally, in these situations, the insurance company will stipulate how long the patient is able to receive therapy. For instance, they might say 30 visits or not to exceed 8 weeks. It is, however, important to know that the procedure for choosing your short-term goals is virtually the same across work settings and various lengths of treatment. The bottom line is that you need to think about how many short-term steps the client can realistically accomplish in the time frame allotted (semester, school year, a month in a rehabilitation hospital, or a week in acute care.)

Another important issue to consider is that most often a client will have more than a single short-term goal. Short-term goals often interlock with one another and they represent different facets of the same underlying aspect of client growth. For example, a child who has a limited expressive lexicon of 40 words at age 3 might have a short-term objective (STO) of increasing lexicon size to 75 words. This client might also have a STO of increasing mean length of utterance (MLU) from 1.0 to 2.0. To increase this MLU, specific types of word combinations might be targeted such as basic operations of reference (more + X, that + X, allgone + X) and two-term semantic relations (agent + action; action + object). Thus, this child has several STOs that involve increasing expressive lexicon size, increasing MLU, increasing use of basic operations of reference, and increasing use of certain two-term semantic relations. When you think about it, all four STOs relate to teaching the child to use multiword utterances. All of this could potentially be accomplished in a university setting during the course of one semester.

WHAT IS A BEHAVIORAL OBJECTIVE?

A behavioral objective is a statement that describes the intended target behavior in an observable and measurable way. The behavioral objective is the staple of everyday treatment planning. Think of the behavioral objective as an instruction manual or a blueprint for how to conduct a therapy session. Just as with building a house, it is difficult to get started without the blueprint. Similarly, without the instruction manual, you would not know how to put together a bookcase, for example, or a child's swing set. You must have a plan for how to conduct a therapy session, and your objectives are your plan. Those objectives not only dictate your behavior in the treatment session but also how you talk and write about what you do in professional communication.

The first thing to remember about objectives is they must be observable and measurable. In order to accomplish this, the clinician must identify what the client is expected to do, under what conditions, and with what degree of success. Owens, Metz, and Haas (2000, p. 143) suggest that the letters ABCD are helpful in remembering the format for writing behavioral objectives:

A. **Audience:** Who is expected to demonstrate the behavior?
B. **Behavior:** What is the observable and measurable behavior?
C. **Condition:** What is the context or condition of the behavior?
D. **Degree:** What is the targeted degree of success?

With this "blueprint" you should be able to write a measurable objective for any behavior that you wish to target in therapy. For example:

A. Billy
B. will spontaneously produce /s/
C. in the initial position of words while naming pictures
D. with 90% accuracy

The following is an example of a language goal:

A. Susan
B. will include narrative elements of setting and character
C. by correctly producing a spontaneous story in response to sequence pictures
D. on 3 out of 5 opportunities during a therapy session

As long as you have identified your client's deficits, based on a thorough assessment, you should be able to apply this formula to create appropriate objectives for treatment. Note that in the above examples we have specified the stimulus (pictures), the task (spontaneous) and the response (/s/ phoneme in words; story production). These are critical components to include in objectives.

Selected words to *avoid* in writing behavioral objectives:

Understand, listen, enjoy, think, know, review, develop an appreciation, like, comprehend, feel, learn, become able, attain, grasp, memorize, acquire, discover, discern, assimilate, digest, grasp, perceive, recognize

We suggest avoiding such words because they are *not measurable and observable.*

Selected words that may be useful in writing behavioral objectives:

> Define, describe, identify, label, list, match, name, outline, select, state, explain, give example, paraphrase, summarize, compute, predict, produce, show, solve, use, diagram, differentiate, discriminate, distinguish, illustrate, outline, select, categorize, compose, organize, plan, rewrite, write, tell, compare, contrast, justify, interpret, ask, choose, follow directions, give, locate, point to, sit, reply, take turns, answer, comply, greet, perform, read, initiate, share, work, combine

WHAT IS A RATIONALE?

One of the most important questions you can ever ask yourself, in any situation, is "Why do I do what I do?" This is certainly true in the field of SLP with intervention planning. Establishing a rationale for your treatment protocol is extremely important, possibly one of the most important aspects of your training. So, that being said, let's talk about rationales and how they are used in therapy.

Webster's dictionary defines *rationale* as "an underlying principle." If you look up the word *rationale* in a thesaurus, you will see words such as *justification, basis, validation, reasoning,* and *logic.* As this applies to speech-language treatment, you must have a basis, or reasoning, for what you do with your clients. The rationale for your treatment may be based upon several factors, most of which come about through ongoing research—there is scientific evidence that proves various treatment techniques are effective. Evidence-based practice (EBP) is a "hot button" issue in our field at this time, and you will most likely hear this term referred to frequently throughout your professional career (Haynes & Johnson, 2009). In 2004, ASHA's executive board stated that the goal of EBP is the integration of: (a) clinical expertise, (b) best current evidence, and (c) client values to provide high-quality services reflecting the interests, values, needs, and choices of the individuals we serve (ASHA, 2004).

In essence, all of the therapy techniques that are being used today, regardless of the specific area (voice, fluency, articulation, language, swallowing, etc.), are used because there is at least some research evidence that shows these techniques are effective. In cases where research evidence is lacking, we should at least be able to provide a theoretical justification for what we decide to do in treatment. This is where the two components of your graduate program, academic and clinical, come together. In your academic training, you will gain the foundational knowledge of each disorder, which includes, but is not limited to, theoretical bases for communication disorders, assessment protocols, and various treatment techniques. You will also become familiar with the research that backs it up. Once you have knowledge of the nature of disorders and assessment/treatment techniques that have been proven effective by research, you can begin to apply it to your clinical preparation (see Figure 5–1). Based on the previous definition of EBP, it only makes sense that you would use this information in planning your treatment, regardless of the setting to which you are assigned for practicum.

All settings, no matter how disparate they might appear at first glance, require practitioners to state goals and objectives, and these statements are always in written form. The following sections are designed to illustrate how goals and objectives are similar yet slightly different across work/practicum settings.

THE UNIVERSITY CLINIC

Most of you will begin your practicum experience in a university clinic. It is for this reason that throughout this book, we will include examples of what forms and reports might look like in this setting. In the university setting, your paperwork requirements are more than in any other practicum environment. As we said in an earlier chapter, the intensity of the university setting in making you state rationales, goals, and objectives and write detailed reports is a valuable learning experience. As a beginning clinician in the university clinic, you may be asked to write a rationale for each goal you develop, and even though you won't continue to do this, it is good practice when you are first starting out. It teaches you how to think about clinical work and enables you to explain your approaches in any amount of detail required. If you gain experience writing behavioral objectives from scratch in the university clinic, you will have a lot less trouble dealing with the check boxes on a form in a medical setting or using a goal bank in a school system. Again, the important thing is the thought process and understanding *why* you choose to work on certain goals as a pathway to helping your client.

With the guidance of clinical supervisors you will find that the university clinic is an excellent setting in which you can learn the "ins and outs" of becoming a competent speech-language clinician. Because a university clinic traditionally operates on a semester by semester basis, your long-term and short-term goals are influenced by this time frame. You may find, however, that long-term goals do not vary much among settings. This is due to the fact that a long-term goal is not usually determined by a specific amount of time (unless in certain medical facilities). It is helpful to remember that a long-term goal is the ultimate change that you want to occur, and it is not always clear as to how long this will take or even if it will ultimately be achieved. What will vary, however, are your short-term goals and how they are written. We will now examine what long-term and short-term goals might look like in the university clinic.

The Integration of Long-Term Goals (LTG), Short-Term Objectives (STO), and Rationales

Because you will see a number of different disorders across the life span in the university clinic, goals may be written many different ways. As mentioned previously, using the ABCD formula may be helpful when writing objectives, even when the objective is written in a simple sentence. Below you will find examples of long-term goals with a short-term objective (STO) for that goal and a rationale for each goal.

Client 1: 3-year-old male

Diagnosis: Limited expressive lexicon, normal receptive vocabulary, only uses single-word utterances (MLU 1.0).

LTG 1: The client will improve receptive and expressive language skills to an age-appropriate level in order to express wants and needs.

STO 1: (A) The client (B) will increase his expressive lexicon size to 75 (C) in spontaneous and imitative naming (D) at home and in clinical sessions as measured by sampling and parent reporting on a lexicon checklist.

Rationale: Two-word utterances are typically not produced by normally-developing children until the lexicon size exceeds 50 (Nelson, 1973).

STO 2: (A) The client (B) will increase MLU to 2.0 (C) in spontaneous and imitative samples (D) taken at 2-week intervals during the semester, at home, and in the university clinical setting.

Rationale: Brown's stages of language development (Brown, 1973) indicate that a 3-year-old child should have a MLU of 2.5 to 3.9.

STO 3: (A) The client (B) will increase production of the basic operations of reference (nomination + X, recurrence + X, and nonexistence + X), (C) in spontaneous and imitative samples, (D) taken at 2-week intervals during the semester, at home and in the university clinical setting.

Rationale: Brown (1973) reported that the first types of word combinations seen in normal development are the basic operations of reference.

STO 4: (A) The client (B) will increase the production of the two-term semantic relations of agent + action and action + object, (C) in spontaneous and imitative samples, (D) taken at 2-week intervals during the semester at home and in the university clinical setting.

Rationale: Brown (1973) reported that agent + action and action + object are early developing semantic relations and they are the basis for SVO constructions.

Client 2: 22-year-old female

Diagnosis: Bilateral vocal nodules

LTG 1: The client will improve voice quality by reducing hoarseness in conversational speech using the facilitative technique of Anterior Focus.

STO: (A) The client (B) will reduce hoarseness using Anterior Focus (C) at the imitative phrase level while reading (D) as measured by a subjective voice quality rating scale administered by the clinician.

Rationale: Anterior or forward focus of the voice results in less abuse of the vocal folds and improved resonance (Boone, McFarlane, & Von Berg, 2005).

Client 3: 5-year-old female

Diagnosis: Articulation disorder

LTG 1: The client will produce age-appropriate phonemes in all positions in conversation with 90% accuracy.

STO 1: The client will produce /k/ initial at the imitative word level with 90% accuracy over six therapy sessions.

STO 2: The client will produce /k/ final at the imitative word level with 90% accuracy over six therapy sessions.

STO 3: The client will produce /k/ medial at the imitative word level with 90% accuracy over six therapy sessions.

Rationale: According to Smit et al. (1990), 90% of females have acquired /k/ by the time they are 3 years, 6 months old; /k/ is an early developing phoneme.

Client 4: 22-year-old male

Diagnosis: Fluency disorder

LTG 1: The client will utilize appropriate fluency shaping techniques and strategies to increase verbal fluency in academic and social settings.

STO: The client will demonstrate using Easy Onset while initiating short phrases on 8 out of 10 trials.

Rationale: Many people who stutter have difficulty on the initial word in an utterance;

the Easy Onset or Easy Relaxed Approach (ERA) technique has proven very effective in initiating speech (Gregory, 2003).

Client 5: 33-year-old male

Diagnosis: English as a second language (ESL); difficulty with pronunciation of English phonemes

LTG 1: The client will improve his use of Standard American English (SAE) in order to communicate more effectively in vocational and social settings.

STO 1: The client will correctly discriminate between minimal pairs /b/ and /v/ when provided with auditory stimuli for 80% accuracy.

STO 2: The client will correctly produce /v/ imitatively in the initial word position during a picture naming task with 80% accuracy.

Rationale: Van Riper and Emerick (1984) recommend that discrimination training occur prior to production training during the establishment phase of treatment; in addition, Locke (1980) states that only error sounds should be included in speech sound discrimination training.

Appendix H shows an example of a university clinic treatment plan.

MEDICAL SETTINGS

Setting goals in medical facilities is somewhat different from that in the university clinic, mainly due to the requirements of health care providers and insurance companies, or third party payers. Any patient who receives speech therapy services in a medical facility will more than likely be covered by an insurance plan or plans (if he has private insurance in addition to Medicare or Medicaid). According to Consumer Driven Health Care (CDHC), a third party payment can be defined as "an insurer paying providers directly for services rendered to the insured, as opposed to an indemnity contract which pays the insured person for losses incurred" (CDHC, 2008).

All health care facilities in the United States are governed by federal laws that regulate how payments are made, the codes used for billing, and the amount of time a patient can receive services. The Centers for Medicare and Medicaid Services (CMS) have the most updated information on Medicare billing procedures and regulations. You can find them on the Web at: http://www.cms.hhs.gov.

When requesting payment from a third party payer for speech therapy services, the speech-language pathologist has to enter a billing code that corresponds with the patient's diagnosis and/or treatment. Diagnosis codes are published by the World Health Organization and are known as ICD-9-CM codes. This stands for International Classification of Diseases-9th revision (Clinical Modification). You will most likely hear them referred to as ICD-9 codes. Billing codes for treatment, also known as CPT or current procedural terminology codes, are published by the American Medical Association and are used in conjunction with ICD-9 codes. CPT codes, originally intended for physicians, are now used widely by many other practitioners (e.g., SLP, physical therapy, occupational therapy). All clinical documentation in a medical facility must support the codes that are billed. This also determines to some extent how goals are written and carried out in a medical setting.

As is the case in the university clinic, the SLP will first decide on a long-term goal for a patient in a medical facility; however, this is not true for all medical facilities. Some hospitals do not establish long-term goals, simply because a short-term goal is more efficacious. A hospital patient may be in an acute care unit for just a few days. In this case, a long-term goal is not necessary. For rehabilitation hospitals, the patient may be in early recovery and still unstable, so realistic long-term goals may not be that obvious. In addition, a patient may only remain in a rehabilitation hospital for 14 to 45 days.

In writing a long-term goal for a patient in any type of medical facility, several factors must be taken into consideration. The SLP usually writes a long-term goal as a first step in establishing a *plan of care* (POC); however, there must be a written order from a physician requesting an evaluation and treatment for speech. For Medicare patients, the plan of care must not only be established and certified by a physician before treatment begins, it must be recertified

by the physician every 30 or 60 days, depending on the setting (Paul & Hasselkus, 2004). An example of a plan of care is included in Appendix I.

In the following section, we will provide examples of long-term goals as they would be written in a rehabilitation facility, hospital, and extended care setting. Keep in mind that in most medical facilities, there is often a "menu" of long-term goals listed, and the SLP will simply check the appropriate goal; however, as a clinical practicum student, you will be expected to discern which goals will be appropriate for your patients based on the evaluation report.

Rehabilitation Setting

Often in this setting, speech therapy (ST) notes are written on the same page with occupational therapy (OT) and/or physical therapy (PT) notes. At one of the sites that we visited, therapists from all three disciplines wrote their notes on one form. The areas to be targeted along with the patient's current level of functioning in each area were also listed. This provides a template for the therapist to go by when working with the patient. For example:

Communication/Cognitive Parameter	Functional Level
Comprehension	Minimal (4)
Expression	Moderate (3)
Intelligibility	Minimal (4)
Memory	Minimal (4)
Attention	Moderate (3)
Problem Solving/Cognition	Moderate (3)
Swallowing	Independent (7)

As you can see, charting like this is very minimal, and once the SLP fills in the appropriate information, it is used to work from each time he treats a patient. It is assumed that a patient who needs moderate assistance will be targeting the next higher level of independence (minimal assistance) as therapy progresses. The functional levels on the above chart are based on *functional independence measures*, or FIM scores, which are widely used in rehabilitation settings. These were developed by the Uniform Data System for Medical Rehabilitation at the State University of New York at Buffalo. You should know that *functional* is the operative word when writing speech and language goals for any patient, but especially so in the medical setting. To that end, *activities of daily living* (ADLs) are often mentioned in patient goals. At this point it is useful to provide a brief summary of FIM scores that you might see in medical treatment goals. The FIMs are used in medical facilities to gauge initial status of the patient and document progress in areas such as self care, bowel/bladder control, mobility, locomotion, communication, psychosocial adjustment, and cognitive function. These areas are typically rated using a seven-point scale that relates to the levels of assistance required by the patient to perform tasks (Medfriendly, 2008). An example of the scale is as follows:

7—Complete independence (timely, safely)

6—Modified independence (extra time, devices)

5—Supervision (cueing, coaxing, prompting)

4—Minimal assist (performs 75% or more of task)

3—Moderate assist (performs 50 to 74% of task)

2—Maximal assist (performs 25% to 49% of task)

1—Total assist (performs less than 25% of task)

These levels of functioning are also commonly used by physical and occupational therapists; therefore, a PT's notes may look very similar to those of the SLP.

Below you will find a sampling of some long-term goals from a rehabilitation facility. Note that the goals are concise. We will also provide several examples of one short-term goal that might accompany these long-term goals.

Sample Long-Term Goals

At first glance, these goals may seem incomplete, confusing, or rather like a foreign language. Once you see them every day, however, they will begin to make sense and soon will become a regular part of your vocabulary.

- Express basic wants/needs via single words/phrases/gestures/augmentative communication
- Identify and solve basic problems related to ADLs/vocational needs
- Follow simple directions (with or without cues) for ADLs
- Speak intelligibly to caregivers at word/phrase level
- Comprehend reading for paragraph length material
- Maximize verbal expression to clearly express complex thoughts/needs
- Perform oral-motor exercise program independently to maximize strength and ROM of oral musculature for speech/swallowing
- Yes/no reliability to facilitate care
- Write legibly for ADLs (i.e., notes, checks)

As is evident from this list of goals, one of the most important factors in establishing long-term goals for patients in a medical facility is that the patient will be able to resume, to the greatest degree possible, the premorbid lifestyle. Most likely, the goal will be written in an abbreviated form [e.g., ↑ verbal reasoning and problem solving from MAX (2) to MOD (3),] with the "up arrow" meaning increase or improve. In this example, FIM scores are in parentheses.

LTG: Express basic wants and needs via single words/phrases/gestures.

STO: Patient will increase (↑) verbal expression for picture identification from Moderate (MOD-3) to Minimum (MIN-4).

LTG: Identify and solve basic problems related to ADLs/vocational needs.

STO: Patient (pt.) will ↑ verbal reasoning and problem solving from Total-1 to MAX-2.

LTG: Follow simple directions (with or without cues) for ADLs.

STO: Pt. will ↑ following commands from MOD-3 to MIN-4.

LTG: Speech intelligible to caregivers at word/phrase level.

STO: Pt. will ↑ intelligibility at phrase level to MOD-3.

LTG: **Reading comprehension for paragraph length material.**

STO: Pt. will ↑ reading comprehension at sentence level to 90% accuracy.

LTG: Maximize verbal expression in order to clearly express complex thoughts/needs.

STO: Pt. will ↑ descriptive tasks to 50% accuracy.

LTG: Perform oral motor exercise program independently to maximize strength and ROM of oral musculature for speech/swallowing.

STO: Pt. will ↑ completion of OMEs from MIN-4 to SPV-5.

LTG: Yes/no reliability to facilitate care.

STO: Pt. will answer yes/no questions with 80% accuracy.

LTG: Writing legible for ADLs (i.e., notes, checks)

STO: Pt. will ↑ written expression for content at sentence level from MAX-2 to MOD-3.

Hospital Setting

As mentioned previously, the SLP in an acute care setting, such as in a hospital, may not develop long-term goals for patients, simply because the duration of their stay does not warrant them. In this case, the SLP will write one or more short-term goals for the patient, based on the initial evaluation. There will more than likely be a description of the patient's deficits included in the evaluation report, and it will be the job of the SLP to develop short-term goals based on this information. The short-term goals will be very similar to the ones listed above or may also be chosen from a menu of goals on a preprinted form. Often, abbreviations will be used instead of words. Refer to Appendix J for a partial list of common medical abbreviations, but keep in mind that these abbreviations may vary by state and facility. Below is an example of short-term goals for patients in a hospital setting:

Patient 1: 72-year-old (y.o.) male

Primary diagnosis: Aphasia

STO 1: Increase (↑) auditory comprehension of one-step commands to 80% accuracy.

STO 2: Increase auditory comprehension of simple yes/no questions to 80% accuracy.

STO 3: Increase automatic speech to 80% accuracy.

Patient 2: 36 y.o. male

Primary diagnosis: TBI

STO 1: Orient to place and time of day with 100% accuracy.

STO 2: Provide biographical information with 80% accuracy.

STO 3: Follow simple commands with 80% accuracy.

Patient 3: 80 y.o. female

Primary diagnosis: Dysarthria

STO 1: Complete OMEs daily to ↑ oral strength and agility.

STO 2: ↑ speech intelligibility at phrase level to MIN-4.

STO 3: ↑ STM to MIN-4.

Note that abbreviations are often used in a hospital setting, as well. In these examples, OME stands for *oral motor exercises*, and STM for *short-term memory*. An up arrow could mean "improve" or "increase."

Patients usually do not remain in an acute care setting for an extended period of time, and your goal, if you are the SLP who is treating this patient, is to figure out what will be most beneficial to this patient during his stay in acute care. This is based on information collected during the patient's evaluation, input from the family (when appropriate), and the patient's prognosis. Refer to Appendix I for more examples of goal writing in a rehab hospital setting.

Long-Term Care/Nursing Home

Long-term care (LTC), *extended care, skilled nursing facility* (frequently referred to as SNIFF), and *nursing home* are names that apply to a facility that provides a range of health, personal care, social, and housing services to people who are unable to care for themselves independently. The SLP who works in one of these facilities will perform many of the same services as an SLP in a hospital or rehabilitation setting; the main difference is the duration of services provided, and this is determined in large part by Medicare.

Any student who has a practicum experience in a LTC facility will become familiar with Medicare, and the terms *Part A* and *Part B*. For the purpose defined in this text, you will not need to have a detailed knowledge of Medicare and its components; however, it is important to know that patients are billed either under Part A or Part B, depending on their age, diagnosis, and length of stay in the facility. Patients who are considered *acute* and are receiving skilled nursing, usually in the first 100 days following their move from the hospital to the LTC facility, are billed under Part A. Patients who are considered more *chronic* and have been in the LTC facility for more than 100 days are billed under Part B (i.e., a patient suddenly begins having difficulty swallowing and is referred to the SLP for evaluation and treatment, even though he has been in the LTC facility for 8 months).

Another reason we mention Part A and Part B in this section is that the requirement for progress notes is different for each one: for Part A, the SLP will complete a weekly note, and for Part B he will complete a daily note. Because most patients in a LTC facility are covered by Medicare, this billing system is the driving force behind how therapy is carried out as well as how all of the supporting paperwork is completed.

Let's examine what goals may look like in a long-term care or nursing home setting. Some LTC facilities provide a "goal bank" for long-term and short-term goals. The following are some examples of long-term goals for dysphagia, which is a fairly common diagnosis for a patient in one of these facilities.

Long-term goals would include:

- Patient will increase oral motor and laryngeal strength and motility to enable efficient oral stage abilities with _____% accuracy.

- Patient will improve ability to adequately self-monitor swallowing skills and perform appropriate compensatory techniques with _____% accuracy.
- Patient will facilitate safe swallowing skills with least restrictive diet via use of compensatory strategies, diet modifications, and caregiver/family education with _____% accuracy.

Short-term goals would be:

- Patient will perform lingual tasks (_____ reps; _____ sets) with _____% accuracy.
- Patient will perform labial tasks (_____ reps; _____ sets) with _____% accuracy.
- Patient will perform bolus manipulation tasks (_____ reps; _____ sets) with _____% accuracy.

These particular short-term goals are written so that the SLP can individualize them for each patient (fill in the blanks as needed), although goals in a LTC setting may not always be written in this way. Two things are usually true regarding goals for patients in a medical setting: (a) they are meant to be functional and (b) they are written in order to restore the patient, to the greatest extent possible, to his prior level of functioning.

PUBLIC SCHOOL SETTING

Any student who completes a speech pathology clinical practicum in the public schools will encounter the *individualized education plan*, or IEP. For any students who have an opportunity to serve children ages birth to 3 years, whether in a preschool, Head Start, or Early Intervention program, the *individualized family services plan*, or IFSP, will also become familiar. In order for you to understand treatment planning and goal-setting in the public school environment, we need to provide some background. It is important for you to know that school systems operate the way they do not because of arbitrary decisions made by school districts, but due to the existence of many complex layers of federal and state law.

Individualized Education Plan (IEP)

The IEP is a written plan outlining the special education program and/or other services (speech therapy) required by a particular student. It identifies learning expectations that are modified from or alternative to the expectations for the appropriate grade and subject, including measurable goals and benchmarks for each goal. It also identifies any accommodations or modifications needed to assist the student in achieving his learning expectations. In addition, the IEP provides a framework for monitoring and reporting progress to parents.

Every student who has been identified as eligible for special education services of any kind must have an IEP. This applies to students who receive speech therapy as a part of other special education services, as well as to students who are served through the general education curriculum and are pulled out for speech therapy.

To create an effective IEP, parents, teachers, administrators, other related services personnel, and sometimes even the student must come together to determine unique needs. These individuals must design an educational program that will help the student be involved in the general curriculum to the greatest extent possible and make educational progress.

The Individuals with Disabilities Education Act (IDEA) requires certain information to be included in each child's IEP; however, states and local school systems often include additional information in IEPs in order to meet federal or state laws. The flexibility that states and school systems have to design their own IEP forms is one reason why IEP forms may look different across school systems or states (United States Department of Education [DOE], 2008).

No Child Left Behind (NCLB) was passed on January 8, 2002, and also impacted the operation of school systems. NCLB is built on four principles: (a) accountability for results, (b) more choices for parents, (c) greater local control and flexibility, and (d) an emphasis on doing what works based on scientific research. We will not entertain a detailed discussion regarding NCLB in this book; however, we will state that due to the realignment of IDEA with NCLB, there now are certain guidelines that all school systems must follow regarding the IEP.

The IEP Development Process

As mentioned previously, the IEP is a written description of an appropriate instructional program for a student with special needs. In order to understand IEP goals, it is useful to know how an IEP is generated. One major difference is that the IEP is developed by a multidisciplinary team of professionals, so the SLP is not writing goals in a vacuum. There are six steps that must be followed in the process of establishing an IEP for any student:

1. **Prereferral:** This is an informal process that involves the classroom teacher identifying the student's educational problems and suggesting solutions. These interventions are attempted for a 6-week period.

2. **Referral:** If the interventions put in place during the prereferral are not successful, then a referral to special education is made. It should be noted that only those students with academic performance extensively behind that of their classmates and/or those who exhibit learning, emotional, and behavioral difficulties can be officially referred. Once the referral is made, an IEP team is created. This team consists of the student's parent(s)/guardian, special education teacher, one general education teacher, and any other professionals who may need to provide services to the student.

3. **Evaluation:** Once the referral has been made, the student must be evaluated to determine if a disability exists, whether special education is required, and, if so, what types of special or related services are needed. The type of evaluation that is performed will be based on the deficits identified during the prereferral and referral processes. Tests may be administered to assess learning, communication, behavior, or a combination of modalities. Federal law mandates that the IEP team must use at least two formal assessments, and that these assessments take place in the student's native language in order to make a determination of eligibility for special education. The team has 60 days from the referral date to determine eligibility.

4. **Eligibility:** Once the results of the evaluation are prepared, the IEP team will meet to determine if

the student meets eligibility requirements. There must be a unanimous decision by the team for the student to be referred for special education services.

5. **Development of an IEP:** Following eligibility determination, the team will decide on the appropriate services and placement for the student, preferably in the least restrictive environment (LRE). A broad definition of LRE is an educational setting where a child with disabilities can receive a free appropriate education designed to meet his or her needs while being educated with peers without disabilities in the regular education environment to the maximum extent appropriate. It is during this phase of IEP development that specific goals are generated. We will discuss this specifically in the next section.

6. **Annual Review:** The IEP team is responsible for conducting an annual review to ensure that the student is meeting goals and/or making progress on the benchmarks specified for each objective that was developed by the team. This review takes place on a yearly basis; however, if the IEP needs to be modified or otherwise updated, a meeting may be called at any time, by any member of the IEP team, to make these revisions.

Components of the IEP

Now that we have discussed the steps involved in creating the IEP, we will outline the specific components, along with the purpose for each. One thing that is important to keep in mind regarding IEPs is that even though they must contain the same basic information, the format may look different from state to state. In researching information from various regions across the country, we found that many states provide copies of their IEP forms on the state's department of education Web site. What we also found is that with a few exceptions, most of the forms follow roughly the same format. Thus, although the IEP format will vary within and across states, there are standard criteria that must be included, regardless of where the document is being written. The IEP will contain the following basic components:

■ **Student Profile/Present Level of Educational Performance (PLEP):** This section outlines biographical data on the student, how the student is performing academically, and a description of the student's speech and/or language deficits.

■ **Progress Reporting:** The IEP states how parents are to be informed of the student's progress, including frequency (at least as often as nondisabled students) and method, whether written reports, phone calls, or conferences.

■ **Special Instructional Factors:** This section is for the purpose of identifying if the student has any limitations that will impede his learning, such as hearing or visual impairment, limited English proficiency, the need for assistive technology, or adaptive physical education.

■ **Transition Services:** This section is designed to address the needs of students in high school in order to implement programs that will enable them to transition from school to a vocational setting or post-secondary education (the age of transition varies from state to state, and can start as early as 14 years). Transition information must address the following areas: (a) recreation and leisure; (b) community participation; (c) post-secondary training and learning opportunities; (d) home living; and (e) work (job and job training).

■ **Transfer of Rights:** This section informs the parent/student that all rights pertaining to special education services transfer to the student at age 18 years. The date the student was notified of the transfer of rights must be indicated in this section of the IEP. Parents must be given a *Notice of Transfer of Parental Rights.*

■ **Goals:** These include broad statements that describe what a student can reasonably be expected to accomplish within a 12-month period of time in a special education program. Goals focus on skills or behaviors, must be related to the child's PLEP, and must be measurable. They must include the student's present level and expected level of performance.

■ **Benchmarks:** Also known as objectives, benchmarks are measurable, intermediate steps leading to the attainment of the goal. There must be at least two benchmarks per goal, and they must include the following: skill/behavior, conditions, criteria, and evaluation methods similar to our earlier discussion of behavioral objectives.

- **Special Education and Related Services:** In this section you will find the type of service being provided (speech therapy) and the anticipated frequency, duration, location, and beginning and ending date of services. This section will also include, if necessary, supplementary aids and services, accommodations needed for assessments, assistive technology, and any other related services.
- **Extended School Year (ESY):** The term *extended school year* encompasses a range of options in providing programs in excess of the traditional 180-day school year, due to issues of regression (loss of skills during an absence of intervention) and recoupment (recovering skills that were lost). In most cases, the IEP team will meet to determine if a student is eligible for ESY and make the appropriate recommendations.
- **Least Restrictive Environment (LRE):** Refers to the amount of time a student with a disability will participate in the regular classroom with nondisabled peers. An explanation of when and why the student will be excluded from the regular classroom is required.
- **Signature section:** The signature of everyone in attendance at the IEP meeting, or who will participate in carrying out the student's IEP, is found in this section. There are generally specific titles listed, such as parent, local educational agency (LEA) representative, special education teacher, general education teacher, student, and other agency representative. There is space for other names to be added, if necessary.

Individualized Family Services Plan (IFSP)

The IFSP came about as a result of *The Program for Infants and Toddlers with Disabilities,* or Part C of IDEA. Part C is a federal grant program that assists states in operating a comprehensive statewide program or early intervention services for infants and toddlers with disabilities, serving children from birth through age 2 years and their families. The program was originally established by Congress in 1986 in recognition of "an urgent and substantial need" to enhance the development of infants and toddlers with disabilities; reduce educational costs by mini-mizing the need for special education through early intervention; minimize the likelihood of institution-alization and maximize independent living; and enhance the capacity of families to meet their child's needs. Children served under Part C of IDEA are those with developmental delay "as measured by appropriate diagnostic instruments and procedures" including: (a) cognitive development; (b) physical development, including vision and hearing; (c) communication development; (d) social or emotional development, and (e) adaptive development (IDEA, 2004). An IFSP documents and guides the early intervention process for children with disabilities and their families. It is the vehicle through which effective early intervention is implemented in accordance with Part C of the IDEA. It contains information about the services necessary to facilitate a child's development and enhance the family's capacity to facilitate the child's development. Through this process, family members and service providers work as a team to plan, implement, and evaluate services tailored to the family's unique concerns, priorities, and resources (IDEA, 2004).

How Is the IFSP Different from the IEP?

There are several factors that distinguish the IEP from the IFSP, but the first and most noticeable difference is the inclusion of the word *family*. The name *individualized family service plan* was chosen because the family is the constant in a child's life and is therefore the focus of the intervention plan. According to the Council for Exceptional Children, there are several ways in which the IFSP differs from the IEP:

- It includes outcomes targeted for the family, as opposed to focusing only on the eligible child.
- It includes the notion of natural environments, which encompass home or community settings. This focus creates opportunities for learning interventions in everyday routines and activities, rather than only in formal, contrived environments.
- It includes activities undertaken with multiple agencies beyond the scope of Part C (see explanation below). These are included to integrate all services into one plan.
- It names a service coordinator to help the family during the development, implementation, and evaluation of the IFSP.

The family's concerns, priorities, and resources guide the entire IFSP process. Early intervention should be seen as a system of services and supports available to families to enhance their capacity to care for their children.

There are also several ways that the IFSP is similar to the IEP. As noted in the section on the IEP, you will find that an IFSP also has the following:

- A statement of the child's present levels of development
- A statement of the family's strengths and needs related to enhancing the child's development
- A statement of major outcomes expected to be achieved for the child and family
- The criteria, procedures, and time lines for determining progress
- The specific early intervention services necessary to meet the unique needs of the child and the family, including the frequency, intensity, and method of delivery
- The natural environment(s) in which services will be provided, including justification, if any, of why the services will not be provided in a natural environment
- The projected dates for initiation of services and their anticipated duration
- Name of the service provider who is responsible for implementing the plan and coordinating with other agencies
- Steps to support the child's transition to preschool or other appropriate services

One thing that you can see from the above goals of the IFSP is the importance of goal-setting. Note that it mentions specific objectives, ways to measure them, and who will measure progress. Appendix K provides an example of an IFSP.

How Does the IEP Reflect Specific Goals?

Any child who has an IEP will have specific annual goals and benchmarks to go along with those goals for every area in which he is receiving special education services, such as reading, math, language, speech.

You may be asking yourself, what is an annual goal? What is a benchmark? These and other questions will be answered in this section, as we explore the world of goal writing in the public schools.

We have been talking about long-term and short-term goals and up until this point have not mentioned anything about benchmarks. The reason for this is that the term *benchmark* is relative only to IEP paperwork. To provide a brief definition, *benchmarks are major milestones that specify skill or performance levels a student needs to accomplish toward reaching his annual goal.* You might be thinking that this is similar to the definition of a short-term goal, and you are exactly correct. Depending on the state, either benchmarks or short-term goals or both are used interchangeably on the IEP. For example, according to the Nebraska Department of Education Web site, a benchmark represents the actual content or performance the student is to accomplish at a specific interval or grade level. It defines a short-term objective as a measurable, intermediate step between a student's present level of educational performance (PLEP) and the annual goals established for the student (Nebraska, 2006). In the State of New Mexico, the goals page is titled, "Annual Goals and Short-Term Objectives or Benchmarks." In Tennessee, the same page is titled, "Measurable Annual Goals and Benchmarks/Short-term Instructional Objectives for IEP/Transition Activities," and in California, the page is simply titled, "Annual Goals and Objectives." See Appendix L for an example of an IEP. Keep in mind that there are software programs that generate IEPs, and many school systems use these. Based on state requirements, school system policies, and how goals are written, you will simply fill in the student's information, and the IEP will be generated for you.

Both benchmarks and short-term objectives are developed based on a logical breakdown of the annual goal and guide the development and modification, as necessary, of strategies that will be most effective in realizing the goals. Goals provide a system for measuring the student's progress toward long-range expectations. After the IEP team develops measurable goals for a student, it must develop effective strategies to realize those goals and measurable, intermediate steps (short-term objectives) or major milestones (benchmarks) that enable families, students, and educators to monitor progress.

Let's take a look at some examples of benchmarks:

1. The student will prepare verbal, written, and visual compositions that fulfill different purposes (to inform, to persuade, to narrate, to entertain).
2. The student will identify and use appropriate language in different settings (school, home, community).
3. The student will understand place value up to three-digit numbers.

Examples of short-term objectives include:

1. David will write answers to simple addition facts with sums 0 to 20 (4 + 5) in 5 minutes on a worksheet at a rate of 40 digits correct per minute with no errors by October 2009.
2. Given different board games and two to three peers, Mary will play cooperatively for 15 consecutive minutes for 10 turn-taking exchanges.

Below you will find some examples of annual goals and benchmarks from two different states. We will start with each student's present level of educational performance (PLEP) and then include annual goals and benchmarks to support the annual goal.

Student 1

PLEP: John exhibits difficulties putting his thoughts on paper. He is very creative but does not understand sentence construction or how to develop paragraphs. He needs to use punctuation and capitalization consistently. John received 12 out of 50 points on the district's assessment for expressive writing. He needs to learn to write the four different sentence types (simple, compound, complex, compound-complex) correctly and integrate them into a paragraph.

Measurable Annual Goal: In 36 weeks John will write at least a six-sentence paragraph using at least three different sentence types scoring 45/50 on the writing rubric.

Benchmarks:

1. John will write simple sentences.
2. John will write compound sentences.
3. John will write complex sentences.
4. John will write compound-complex sentences.

Student 2 (from a different state)

PLEP: David is a 4-year-old male who lives with his parents and two older brothers. He attends a preschool at his church three times per week. His teacher reports that he interacts well with his peers at preschool. She also indicated on a checklist that David is more difficult to understand than the other children in the class and does not use sentences as long as those of the other children. He has a history of ear infections and has had two sets of PE tubes placed in his ears. He is reported to also have trouble with allergies and infrequent episodes of asthma. Phoneme production deficits adversely affect phonological awareness and his limited expressive skills restrict his participation in oral classroom activities and social interaction in the preschool environment. Standardized testing revealed reduced vocabulary development and mean length of utterance (MLU). He cannot answer questions appropriately. His articulation errors are developmentally inappropriate for a child his age and cause his speech to be difficult to understand to both familiar and unfamiliar listeners. David becomes easily frustrated when not understood.

Measurable Annual Goal: By May 2008, David will verbally express himself by using four- to five-word sentences while asking/answering "wh" questions 8/10 trials in structured conversational analysis.

Benchmarks:

1. By the end of the first 9 weeks, David will answer "who" and "what" questions using stories and pictures as stimuli with 80% accuracy.
2. By the end of the second 9 weeks, David will answer "where" and "when" questions using stories and pictures as stimuli with 80% accuracy.
3. By the end of the third 9 weeks, David will ask "who" and "what" questions using books, pictures, and orally read stories as stimuli with 80% accuracy.

Measurable Annual Goal: David will eliminate use of final consonant deletion by producing the target phonemes /p,m,n,b,k,g,d,t/ in the final position with 90% accuracy in structured oral activities in his preschool classroom as measured by SLP progress monitoring.

Benchmarks:
1. By the end of the first 9 weeks, David will imitate the target phonemes at the word level with 80% accuracy.
2. By the end of the second 9 weeks, David will produce the target phonemes at the spontaneous word level with 80% accuracy.
3. By the end of the third 9 weeks, David will produce the target phonemes at the spontaneous phrase/sentence level with 80% accuracy.
4. By the end of the fourth 9 weeks, David will produce the target phonemes in structured oral activities with 90% accuracy.

As you can see, goals, benchmarks, and objectives are written quite differently across states, and it will be up to you to familiarize yourself with your school's process. What is also important to consider is that goals, benchmarks, and objectives must be written so they can pass the "stranger test." In other words, they should be written so that someone who did not write them could use them to develop appropriate instructional plans and assess student progress. They should also be written to pass the "so what test," meaning the IEP team considers the importance of the goal, objective, or benchmark. The team would pose the question, "Is the skill indicated in this goal, objective, or benchmark really an important skill for the student to learn?" If the answer is "No," then most likely, the goal isn't appropriate. In many ways, this is similar to the functional goals targeted in medical environments with adults. For children, the ability to function in the school environment is an important aspect of their lives.

SIMILARITIES AND DIFFERENCES IN GOAL-WRITING ACROSS WORK SETTINGS

Figure 5–2 illustrates goal writing similarities and differences across university, medical, and educational settings. Let's first remind you about similarities. First

of all, every work setting requires that goals are set and that they are written down in some format. Second, the goals must be measurable and thus written to some degree as behavioral objectives. A third similarity is that in all settings the SLP is required to take periodic measurements to determine if the client is making progress toward the goal that was initially set. Fourth, documentation is viewed as critical in all work settings. Finally, the functional relevance of goals is important in all work settings. While a student in a university clinic could write a goal that was not particularly functional, it is always ideal to develop goals that are functionally relevant. Obviously, in medical settings functional goals are mandated, and in educational settings, academic relevance is paramount.

Goal-setting differences across work settings revolve around several issues. First, there can be more or less involvement of multidisciplinary teams in developing goals. This is more important in medical and school settings than in the university clinic. The place where goals are written down is a second difference among settings. In the university setting, we write goals in treatment plans or reports that are placed in a client's folder. In medical settings, the goals are part of a patient's medical chart. In school systems, the IEP is the place to write goals. A third difference in goal writing is the length and form of the goal statements. In the university setting, goals are written in narrative form and tend to be lengthier than in other settings. In the medical setting, goals are brief and there is liberal use of medical abbreviations. Goals in school systems are often midway between university and medical settings in length. A fourth difference among settings is the length of the sample gathered to verify progress toward goals. In the university, it is not unusual for students to take language samples several times during a semester to verify progress. On the other hand, medical settings use short tasks and FIM scores to monitor patient progress. School systems, again, are midway between medical settings and university clinics. They often monitor progress with nonstandardized tasks but also give standardized assessments on an annual basis to see if change has occurred. A fifth difference among settings is the presence of a written rationale for goals. In the university setting, students are given practice in developing rationales as part of their goals when they are first beginning practicum. Rationales are almost never seen in the documentation produced

Goal-Writing Differences Across Work Settings

University	Medical	School
• Not team oriented • Goals written in client folder • Goals may be functional • Goals longer and more descriptive • Procedures are more detailed • More extensive data gathered in samples • Rationale often provided • Goals can be changed quickly • Goals are for semester	• Team oriented • Goals written in patient chart • Goals Must be functional • Behavioral Objectives very brief with abbreviations • Smaller samples gathered • Use of FIM Scores • Wording of goals important for reimbursement • Rationale implied but not written • Goals often for short time periods	• Team Oriented • Goals written on IEP • Goals educationally based • Goals written in medium length • Moderate sized samples • Rationale implied or loosely stated • Difficult to change goals without IEP meeting • Goals are annual with periodic benchmarks

Goal-Writing Similarities Across Work Settings
- **Written goals are required**
- **Goals must be written behaviorally**
- **Periodic measurement is required to determine progress**
- **Documentation of progress is important**
- **Functional relevance of goals is optimal**

Figure 5–2. Similarities and differences of goal writing across work settings.

by medical facilities and school systems. A sixth difference among settings is the ability to easily change goals. In medical facilities the use of reimbursement codes and oversight by the medical establishment may make it difficult to change goals quickly. In the school setting it may require the IEP team to reconvene to discuss changes in objectives. The university clinic can change goals whenever the practicum supervisor feels it is necessary.

It is also important to mention computerized reports again in this section. Not only do software programs generate diagnostic reports; they can also create progress reports, treatment plans, and discharge notes. Depending on the facility, you may find that you are writing reports on your own or that all you do is enter the client data into a computer and the report is generated for you. Either way, you still have to discern what information is pertinent and where to write it. It is our hope that the information in this book is helpful and that you will gain this valuable insight through your clinical practicum experiences. Please refer to the listing in Chapter 4 for some selected software programs.

Our discussion of goal writing has attempted to introduce the practicum student to the elements of well-crafted goals that apply to any work environment. We have also tried to alert students to the changes in goal writing that will be encountered as they do clinical practicum across different types of settings. Hopefully, you will take some comfort in the similarities and view the differences as a challenge and not a threat.

6 Short-Term Progress Reporting

> **Supervisor in medical facility:** "I'm having a hard time understanding what you wrote here about your therapy session. What do all of these numbers mean?"
>
> **Student:** "Well, uh . . . I tried to write down my data so that it makes sense. Why is this so important, anyway? I know he's making progress—isn't that all that matters?"
>
> **Supervisor:** "Of course it matters that he's making progress, but you need to have the right documentation to back it up, especially if we want to get paid!"

Ah, the real world . . . the place where money is the name of the game—at least, that is, if you're talking about the real world of hospitals, nursing homes, or a private practice. Here, billing policies, copayments, insurance claims, and reimbursement are an everyday part of life. Patients must pay for services, and in most cases, their health insurance, whether it's Medicare, Medicaid, or private, will cover the cost.

There are places, however, where this is not the case. Take for instance, the public schools. There, you don't have to worry about establishing fees for your services, filing insurance claims, or methods of payment. And unless you work in a school system that bills Medicaid, you don't have to worry about payments for services at all.

Yes, it is true that in many parts of the real world, you won't get paid if you don't have the adequate documentation to back up what you're doing in therapy. But it's also true that even in the world of the university clinic, which some will claim is not "the real world," you learn to report on your clients' progress because it is an integral part of the therapy process—not just because you won't get paid! You

would think a doctor was crazy if he put you on medication for an infection and then commented, "Well, we just thought we'd try those pills for the heck of it. We don't really care what effect they're having."

Reporting on the progress of your clients and/ or patients is paramount to a successful course of treatment. According to a document found on the ASHA Web site, "Clear and comprehensive records are necessary to justify the need for treatment, to document the effectiveness of that treatment, and to have a legal record of events" (Paul & Hasselkus, 2004). In addition, as cited in Pannbacker, Middleton, Vekovius, and Sanders (2001, p. 39), the ASHA Professional Services Board (ASHA, 1990), which defines standards for clinical service in speech-language pathology, states, "The quality of services provided is evaluated and documented on a systematic and continuing basis . . . " In other words, the only way for you to know if what you are doing in therapy is working is to take accurate data, analyze that data on a daily or weekly basis, and then make modifications accordingly. Otherwise, you are just "tilting at windmills," as the old saying goes.

At this point, you may be asking yourself, "But how will I know how to do this?" For starters, one of the main purposes of this book is to expose you to the paperwork and reporting requirements you will be expected to master by the time you finish your graduate work. That way, when you are called upon to complete any type of reporting function, whether it's related to assessment or treatment, you will at least have an idea of what to expect. In addition, your clinical supervisor(s) will assist you a great deal when you begin your clinical practicum experience. ASHA understands the importance of good supervision when it relates to students in training—so much so, in fact, that it has outlined 13 supervisory "tasks" that inform student clinicians of what to expect from their supervisors. These guidelines insure that all students enrolled in SLP practicum will be guided and directed in all areas of service delivery by a competent, licensed clinician.

DAILY PROGRESS REPORTING

There would be no way to measure the efficacy of your speech-language therapy if not for daily progress reporting. Data that is taken during each therapy session will be used to determine several things: (a) if the patient/client is making progress, (b) that the treatment techniques are appropriate, (c) when modifications need to be made, and (d how to plan for future sessions.

The SOAP note, as it's affectionately known in the world of SLP, is a staple of daily reporting on client progress. *SOAP* is an acronym that stands for *subjective, objective, assessment,* and *plan.* SOAP notes are also commonly used by medical and rehabilitation staff and therefore may appear frequently in other sections of medical charts.

The following is a description of each area of the SOAP note and an example of the information contained therein:

Subjective: A description of the client's physical and/or emotional state, including affect, mood, level of motivation, attention, and so on. It is also appropriate to use direct quotes when warranted.

Example 1: Mr. Jones was in a pleasant mood during therapy today, although he stated that he was a little tired. His wife said, "He didn't sleep well last night." He had difficulty concentrating at times.

Example 2: Cowan was eager to begin therapy today. She told the clinician, "I've been practicing my new /s/ sound!"

Objective: Information regarding the behaviors you targeted in therapy; includes session goals and data for each goal. If testing was done, write the name of the test(s) administered and the results. According to Meyer (2004), *the facts* belong in the objective part of the SOAP note. In addition to your data, you want to include any information that will support a statement made in the subjective part (Meyer, 2004).

Example 1: Client/patient will improve immediate memory by repeating eight-word sentences with 75% accuracy.

Data: Mr. Jones only achieved 40% correct responses, compared to 70% from last week, due to his fatigue and lack of concentration.

Example 2: Client/patient will produce /s/ imitatively at the phrase level with 90% accuracy.

Data: Cowan was 85% accurate today, with very little prompting.

Assessment: Includes an explanation of what your data means, if necessary. Also includes where you would describe how your client performed and discuss factors that may have affected performance.

Example: Client had difficulty with /f/ initial, although she was stimulable for /f/ final in CVC words. There also seems to be a facilitating context, in that she could produce /f/ more easily if it followed the vowels /E/ and /ae/.

Plan: Includes a statement about what is planned for the next treatment session.

Example: Continue to target /f/ initial and final, and probe for stimulability for /f/ in the medial position of single words.

Now that we know what is contained in the SOAP note, let's examine what one will look like across the various settings and how they are used in everyday treatment.

UNIVERSITY CLINIC

As a practicum student in the university clinic, you will serve clients with a variety of diagnoses across the life span. In almost all university clinics, students are taught to use the SOAP note as the primary tool for data reporting. In our clinic, students write a SOAP note for each session, whether the client comes one, two, or three times per week. This may not be the case in all clinics. In other situations, students may write just one note for the week, regardless of how many sessions are included. It should be noted that the SOAP note should be concise and detailed, although abbreviations can be used, and information does not have to be communicated using complete sentences as long as it is understandable to the person reading the note.

In most cases, the SOAP notes are kept in the client's "working file," usually in the clinical supervisor's office, so that the student and supervisor can discuss the client's progress during their weekly supervisory conference. In our clinic, every client has a confidential file that is kept in a locked cabinet in our clinic office. For speech clients, the clinical supervisor keeps a file in her office where daily objectives and SOAP notes are kept, along with a record of the student's clinical hours. This is where all of the daily progress notes are kept, so that they are easily accessible to both student and supervisor.

In some settings, speech-language pathologists (SLPs) fill out weekly and monthly progress reports; however, this is not usually the case in the university clinic. In general, the SOAP notes are used to record all of the data for the semester, and then this information is summarized in the end of semester treatment or progress report. For this reason, information contained in the SOAP note must be timely and accurate. Without accurate data, it is very difficult to determine if true progress is being made. Let's examine a few SOAP notes from clients in the university clinic.

Example 1: Aphasia Client

Subjective: Mr. Smith was pleasant and cooperative today. He put forth good effort throughout the session, except with confrontational naming, which seemed to frustrate him.

Objective: STO 1: The client will spontaneously match pictures with their descriptions from a field of 5 with 80% accuracy.

Data: 79%

STO 2: The client will spontaneously name common household objects with 60% accuracy.

Data: 23%

STO 3: The client will provide the missing word in a common phrase with minimal cues from the clinician with 80% accuracy.

Data: 28%

STO 4: The client will copy the clinician's model of personal/pertinent information with 90% accuracy.

Data: 76%

Assessment: Mr. Smith did very well with matching pictures to their written description. His reading skills continue to improve, although he still struggles with verbal expression. He had a particularly difficult time with confrontational naming today and would give up easily. This may be due to the fact that he did well with this task last week.

Plan: Continue to target expressive language skills; may have to modify goal of confrontational naming due to level of difficulty. Talk to him about using his left hand more often for fine motor tasks other than writing.

Example 2: Child Language Client

Subjective: Max was very active today, and difficult to keep on task. His mother stated, "He has a lot of energy this morning!"

Objective: STO 1: The client will respond appropriately to "what" and "where" questions after listening to a short story with 80% accuracy.

Data: 50% (goal may have been higher had Max been able to stay on task)

STO 2: The client will demonstrate sound-letter recognition from a set of three letters with 80% accuracy.

Data: Max was able to identify four out of six letters (66%) and identify the correct sound for three out of four (75%).

STO 3: The client will read 10 out of 15 possible sight words when presented on flash cards by the clinician.

Data: 8/15 or 53%

Assessment: Max enjoyed the bingo game for reviewing letter-sound recognition. He performed better when he was given the sound and could choose the matching letter. Max's response to cues continues to be inconsistent, although choice cues seem to be the most effective. He tends to lose focus toward the end of the session, so he may require more frequent breaks.

Plan: Continue to work on "what" and "where" questions, using choice cues, and then a complete model when needed. Continue working on letter-sound recognition; have Max match the sound to the letter, and vice versa.

Example 3: Child Articulation Client

Subjective: Hannah was very happy today and ready to begin therapy.

Objective: STO 1: The client will produce /k/ in the initial position of words with 80% accuracy.

Data: 2/12 or 17%

STO 2: The client will produce /f/ in the initial position of words with 80% accuracy.

Data: 4/12 or 33%

Assessment: Hannah had a lot of difficulty producing /k/ initial in words. Even when the clinician used a tongue depressor, mirror, and verbal prompts, she was still only able to produce it correctly 2 out of 12 times. She responds well to stickers and is very motivated by the memory game, so these will be continued as reinforcement.

Plan: Continue with production of /k/ and /f/ initial and probe for /k/ in medial and final word position to determine if there is a facilitating context.

Example 4: Fluency Client

Subjective: Doug was in a good mood today. He was excited about the upcoming spring break.

Objective: STO 1: The client will reduce dysfluencies to less than 20% during 3 minutes of oral reading in the therapy room.

Data: 12% dysfluent (15/123 words) in 4 paragraphs

STO 2: The client will reduce dysfluencies to less than 20% during a 3-minute conversation with a familiar person in the therapy room.

Data: 19% (15/80) in 2 minutes of conversation

STO 3: The client will reduce dysfluencies to less than 20% when speaking to an unfamiliar person in the therapy room.

Data: 26% (100/386) in 10 minutes of conversation

Assessment: Doug's reading was not as fluent as usual. He stated that he did not focus on being "relaxed as he should have." He still felt that "overall, it was pretty good." He had difficulty when speaking with Alex, an unfamiliar person, and admitted that his blocks were longer and more frequent because he wasn't using his techniques.

Plan: Videotape the next session to allow for more feedback; continue to talk to him about his self-monitoring skills.

These are just a few examples of what a SOAP note looks like. As mentioned previously, the SOAP format is used in many different settings and will vary in length, detail, and content, depending on the setting.

MEDICAL SETTINGS

Many of the medical professionals we interviewed informed us that it is often the case that students are timid or hesitant when writing information in a patient's chart. They seem to be afraid of writing the wrong information, writing too much information, or not writing enough information. It is our goal to help you know what to write, and how to write it, so this won't happen to you.

As mentioned previously, SOAP notes are standard documentation for many different medical professionals. In a hospital, nursing home, or rehab hospital, doctors, nurses, and rehab staff (therapists) may all use SOAP notes to communicate regarding a patient's care. Therefore, many of the SOAP notes found in a patient's chart may look similar. What will distinguish a speech-language SOAP note from a medical SOAP note will be the goals that are written in the Objective section. What will distinguish a speech-language SOAP note in a medical facility from a speech-language SOAP note anywhere else is the medical terminology that will be contained therein. We feel it's worth explaining a few terms, abbreviations, and symbols that you may encounter in a medical setting. Appendix J lists the most commonly used symbols and abbreviations and their meaning. Due to the limited amount of space, as well as the number of professionals who add information to a patient's

medical chart, you can appreciate the need for the SLP in a medical setting to use abbreviations and symbols as often as possible.

Depending on the facility, terminology may vary based on the type of system used to measure a patient's progress. As we mentioned in Chapter 5, it is common to see *functional independence measures* or FIM scores. This system, as the name implies, evaluates patients based on their level of independence.

We have found that most facilities use this system or one that is similar. Some facilities may only use the numbers from the FIM scale or similar abbreviations. For instance, they may write, "Pt. will improve from level 4 to level 5," or they may use MOD or MIN rather than MIN-A (minimum assistance) or MOD-I (moderate impairment). In general, the criteria are the same even if the abbreviations vary. Let's take a look at what a SLP note might actually look like in a rehabilitation setting. The following SOAP note is for a patient who was working on memory, intelligibility, and orientation using a functional independence rating.

Subjective: Pt. seen for 30 minutes of speech tx today; pt. alert & cooperative.

Objective: Pt. completed OMEs c̄ SPV, to ↑ ROM. Pt. able to recall 2/3 speech strategies and completed speech intelligibility tasks at sentence level c̄ SPV.

Assessment: Pt. is only requiring min. A with speech intelligibility tasks, but continues to require mod. A with cognitive retraining tasks.

Plan: Continue POC

Due to daily caseload numbers, lack of space in the medical chart, and the number of people who have to read the information, most speech pathology notes in a medical setting are brief and use similar terminology. This is true for other therapists as well as nurses, doctors, and other professional staff, making it even more important that the SLP in a medical setting become familiar with all types of terminology.

Another acronym that you may see in a medical facility (namely, rehabilitation facilities) is what's known as the *inpatient rehabilitation facility—patient assessment instrument* (IRF-PAI). The SLP uses this instrument to assess a patient's current level of functioning, develop goals, measure progress, and determine when a patient is ready to be discharged. Usually, an administrator at the facility will then collect all the data on this patient (from all therapists) and record it on the IRF-PAI form. This form is also required for all Medicare Part A patients in order to determine the number of days that Medicare will approve for in-patient treatment in a rehab facility.

The IRF-PAI rates patients based on a FIM system, but may use different terminology. For example, a Level 5 patient according to this form requires "Standby Prompting," which correlates to Level 6 on the FIM system, which would indicate the patient requires "Supervision."

PUBLIC SCHOOL SETTINGS

Due to the federally mandated use of the individualized education plan (IEP), the SOAP note is not a staple of reporting in the public schools. Most SLPs who work in the public schools devise their own system to track data and simply report final data in the section of the IEP form that is designated specifically for reporting progress. Methods of data collection may vary greatly among school systems, schools within the same system, or individual therapists. As a practicum student in the public schools, you will be expected to follow the system that your particular school has in place. This may mean that you will use specific data collection forms or that you design your own form; each school will be different.

Even though forms and procedures may differ across school systems, what remains the same is how each child's progress is reported on the actual IEP form. This is federally mandated, and therefore not open to interpretation.

We have provided a sample Annual Goal Progress Report form that is used in our local school system (Appendix M). You will notice that there are six reporting periods, as well as a legend in the middle of the page that is used to evaluate the student's progress toward the annual goals. This information is of paramount importance in determining changes to be made to the IEP when it is updated each year and must be documented on the IEP during the designated reporting period. This designated "progress reporting" period may not be the same across school systems. In the State of Alabama, progress must be documented on the student's IEP every 9 weeks; however, your particular school's requirements may be different.

Progress reporting is a necessary component of the delivery of SLP services. Becoming efficient at reporting progress or lack thereof, regardless of the setting in which you eventually practice, is a crucial skill to develop as a student clinician and one that will only enhance your clinical skills throughout your professional career.

7 Long-Term Progress Reports

Our goal as speech-language pathologists is to help our clients/patients attain or return (to the greatest extent possible) normal function of their speech, language, or swallowing abilities. In order to accomplish this task, we must rely on data that measure and validate this change over time. As we have discussed in previous chapters, these data are what determines if we have achieved our goals through the delivery of speech-language pathology services, as well as our ability to receive payment or reimbursement (from a third party payer) for those services. Now that we have shown you how to write goals, objectives, daily notes, and short-term progress reports, we would be remiss if we did not discuss how to report progress for patients who are in therapy for an extended period of time. This chapter will provide setting-appropriate information on long-term progress reports as well as information about discharge summaries, when they are needed, and what they look like.

UNIVERSITY CLINIC

Due to the nature of how treatment takes place in a university clinic, namely, that clients receive treatment for the duration of a quarter or semester, the long-term progress report generally serves as a summary for the therapy term. In addition to the daily SOAP or weekly progress notes, most training programs require students to prepare a final report that includes data for all of the client's goals for the entire term. This document may be referred to as a final treatment report or progress report, depending on the university program and the terminology it chooses to use. Most clients who attend a university clinic for

speech-language services expect these reports, as do other allied professionals who collaborate with clinicians in university clinics.

For example, if a child is receiving services in the public school as well as at the university clinic, a copy of the long-term progress report is usually sent to the school SLP in order to insure that both parties are addressing the same needs for the child. Also, if a child has been referred to the university clinic by another professional (psychologist, physician, occupational therapist, etc.), it is standard practice to send that individual a copy of the client's progress report with a note thanking him for the referral. If a client is being seen by a number of different professionals, this sharing of information can be vital in the overall treatment of the client.

The long-term progress report is important for several reasons, which we will explain below. This may include, but is not limited to:

1. Short-term and long-term progress reporting is required by ASHA and third party payers, when necessary.

   All university programs must abide by certain ASHA guidelines in order to maintain their accreditation. These guidelines stipulate that a variety of documentation must be in place on a consistent basis. Students must keep an accurate record of their clinical hours, and there must be a system in place to keep up with each client's progress. Most clinics have a confidential file system, in which each client has a personal and confidential file that is kept in a secure location. At the end of each term, treatment reports or long-term progress reports must be placed in the client's file for safekeeping. ASHA requires this confidential filing system, as does the federal government, due to enactment of the Health Information Portability and Accountability Act (HIPAA). As far as billing is concerned, if a clinic bills Medicaid, Medicare, or private insurance, accurate records insure that these entities are being billed for valid service delivery. Any discrepancies in paperwork can result in denial of payment for services and this reflects poorly on the program, the clinic, and the university.

2. Clients may remain in therapy for several semesters, or even years, and historical data are important when planning treatment each term.

It is not uncommon for many patients (especially adults) in a university clinic to end up there due to an insurance company being unwilling to continue paying for services through a hospital or private practitioner. As we discussed in an earlier chapter, third party payers usually stipulate the exact number of sessions they will cover relating to any type of rehabilitation therapy. Once the patient has completed the designated number of sessions, he must find services elsewhere or pay out-of-pocket expenses. And, due to the fact that university clinics are training facilities, many operate on a sliding fee scale, based on a client's ability to pay. It is also necessary that students have clients for whom they can provide services in order for the clinical training program to thrive. Therefore, some clients will remain in therapy for an extended period of time due to the reduced fees and willingness of the clinical staff at the university clinic to work with them.

3. Clients often have a new student clinician each semester, depending on the circumstances.

Most university training programs have the goal of providing student clinicians with the most diverse clinical experience possible, allowing them to work with both children and adults in a variety of disorder areas. This is usually accomplished through practicum experience in the university clinic as well as off-campus sites. It is for this reason that clients are often seen in the university clinic that have been discharged from other private practitioners, hospitals, or rehabilitation facilities, due to insurance reasons or lack of progress. Generally, clients in the university clinic will have a new student clinician each semester in order for students to receive training in all disorder areas. This is especially true for a client with a less common disorder.

4. The client and/or parent or caregiver is provided with a record of progress.

Just as you expect a report from a physician or specialist when you have any type of testing or treatment done, your clients expect the same information regarding the speech therapy services you have provided. Not only are clients/parents given progress reports in order to summarize data for themselves or their child's therapy sessions, in the case of older children and adults, the progress report may serve as a tool to motivate the clients to continue with therapy until maximum potential is achieved.

It is important to add here that many times, the long-term progress report will also serve as a discharge summary. If a client is being discharged from therapy, this is usually mentioned in the Recommendations section of the report. For example, "Based on Mr. Smith's excellent progress over the past several weeks, it is recommended that he be discharged from speech therapy at this time." More than likely, your clinic will have protocols in place for how and when to write progress/treatment reports, and your clinical supervisors will assist you in this process. However, we provide an example of a university clinic long-term treatment report in Appendix N.

MEDICAL SETTINGS

Due to the nature of treatment across various medical settings, we will address each one separately in this section.

Rehabilitation Hospital

As we mentioned in Chapter 4, patients are typically admitted to a rehabilitation hospital for a predetermined amount of time. This depends on the patient's level of functioning, often referred to as *burden of care*, as well as their insurance coverage. Persons aged 65 or older are eligible for Medicare, whereas patients under the age of 65 must rely on private insurance or pay expenses out of pocket. The average stay for Medicare patients is 14 days, although patients who have private insurance may stay longer, depending on how much time their insurance company will allow. At the culmination of their stay in the rehabilitation facility, one of three things will happen. They are (a) discharged home, (b) referred back to the hospital, or (c) sent to a long-term care facility.

As was evident in the chapter on writing long-term and short-term goals, some facilities do not even bother to write long-term goals, although others have a long-term goal, but the outcomes reflect what one could reasonably expect to accomplish during a 2-week period. For example, a client in a university clinic may have a long-term goal of returning to work on a part-time basis following a stroke or TBI, whereas this same individual may have a long-term goal of following multi-step directions with minimal assistance while in the rehabilitation facility. You may want to refer back to Chapter 5 for examples of long-term goals for each type of medical facility. The progress report for these patients will reflect not only the goals that were targeted, but also the amount of time the patient spends working on these goals.

A long-term progress report may also serve as the discharge report for a patient who has only spent 14 days in a rehabilitation facility. The discharge summary may be the same form that was used for reporting the patient's progress and will also use functional independence measures (FIM) scores to indicate the patient's status at discharge. At times, the SLP may actually discharge a patient from speech therapy before he is discharged from a facility. If this is the case, you will generally write a *discharge note* on a specific form, sometimes called a *patient status form* or *patient update form*. If applicable, you may be required to complete a specific section labeled "Speech" on an interdisciplinary discharge form. Along with discharge instructions, you may fill out a Patient Education section that indicates what information you have provided to the patient regarding any necessary home care. You will find an example of a progress report/discharge summary from a rehabilitation hospital in Appendix O.

Hospital

Similar to the rehabilitation setting, a patient's stay in a hospital may be very limited. Very often, patients are seen in acute care for just a few days until they are stable enough to be moved to the skilled nursing wing of the hospital or discharged home. As a general rule, patients do not have long-term goals in acute care; it is the goal of the medical professionals working with patients in acute care to get them medically stable so that they can participate in and benefit from any therapies they may need once they recover. The SLP who sees a patient in acute care may be there only to do a bedside swallowing evaluation to determine if the patient is able to eat and drink solid food or if he will need to be tube fed. In many cases, the SLP will not see this patient for any type of speech or language therapy until he has been moved from acute care.

Once the patient has been transferred to another part of the hospital and it has been determined that he may have speech, language, or swallowing problems, the physician will write an order for the SLP evaluation. Once this evaluation has been completed and the patient's needs are determined, the SLP will then write appropriate goals for the patient and begin treatment. You may refer back to Chapter 5 for examples of short-term and long-term goals in a hospital setting. Also, provided in Appendix Q is an example of a speech pathology discharge summary from an acute care hospital.

Long-Term Care Facility/Nursing Home

Unless they have been temporarily transferred to the nursing home until they recover enough function to return home, most patients who are in long-term care may remain there for the duration of their life. Even though these patients may remain in the long-term care facility a very long time, they will only qualify for speech-language therapy for a specific amount of time. Therefore, long-term progress reports for these patients are very similar to those of the acute care or rehabilitation hospital. The SLP often uses appropriate goals from a *goal bank* and then selects short-term objectives as a way to achieve the long-term goal. Once again, goals must be functional in order for the facility to be reimbursed by Medicare or other third party payers—if the patient is not making progress, the case cannot be made that he should continue receiving services. The long-term goal will most likely be written so that it may be achieved in the time frame that has been stipulated by payment for services.

PUBLIC SCHOOLS

If you find yourself assigned to a practicum in the public schools, you will become very familiar with the individualized education plan (IEP). With the information we have provided in Chapter 5, along with the experience you gain first hand, you will begin to develop an understanding of how the IEP functions. The IEP has a built-in system for tracking progress. If you recall from Chapter 5, benchmarks are developed for each long-term goal that stipulate a time frame for each goal to be achieved. Personnel responsible for implementing the IEP must then report the student's progress to the parent or guardian of the child who is receiving services on a regular basis. Due to the nature of this periodic reporting system, there is no long-term progress report for children who are being served through the public schools— progress is reported at various intervals throughout the school year, such as every 6 or 9 weeks, and then the parent(s), teachers, special education teachers, and other professionals meet once a year to discuss how the child has progressed based on the benchmarks set forth from the previous year's meeting. In this way, each person who is responsible for implementing the IEP will understand the ultimate academic goal for this child.

It is probably fairly clear to you now that reporting progress is a mainstay in the field of SLP. Without reports of how our clients are performing, we have no way to determine if we should stay the course, modify treatment, or discharge someone from therapy altogether. The long-term progress report tells us if the long-term goal (the ultimate outcome we want for our clients) is being achieved, and if not, how we should proceed in the future.

8 Professional Correspondence

Although we have discussed many forms of written communication that you will be expected to master during your clinical training, one that we have not addressed is professional correspondence. In the course of a normal work week the speech-language pathologist will generate a variety of different types of correspondence in addition to the report writing we have discussed in previous chapters. Whether you are writing referral letters, transmittal letters, thank-you letters, e-mails, or memoranda, the ability to communicate effectively will speak volumes about your knowledge, clinical competence, organization, and professionalism. In short, you will establish credibility with professional and well-written communication. Professionalism is not just reserved for our verbal interactions and clinical reports; it shows up in our written correspondence as well.

How does your written communication project an image of you? Imagine if you will that you are a parent whose child is receiving speech-language therapy at the university clinic. You receive a letter from the student who has been working with your child, and in the first paragraph, there are two typographical errors and a run-on sentence. What is your impression going to be? Would you think that this student is professional or unorganized? Would you wonder if this graduate student's lack of attention to detail might carry over to her preparation for your child's therapy? We feel the latter would be true. The way we communicate, whether verbally or in writing, truly does say a lot about us as professionals.

During your time in school, you will be required to demonstrate two types of writing: academic and clinical. Academic writing includes research papers, term papers, journal reviews, or even answers to comprehensive test questions. Clinical writing encompasses all of the reports and documents we have covered thus far in this text, in addition to the type of correspondence we address in this chapter—e-mails, referral letters, and the like. Although you are expected to come into the university with some basic writing skills that enable you to complete these academic writing tasks, we understand that clinical writing is a unique genre of communication. Most students will not come into a training program with knowledge of professional clinical writing. This is a skill you will acquire right along with the clinical competencies you develop toward becoming a certified SLP.

THE BASICS

Professional writing is a challenging yet important and necessary part of your training. Lack of student preparedness in training programs is nothing new, however; the authors have learned through interviews with practicum supervisors and in professional seminars that students' writing skills are frequently an area of weakness. In other words, this is a problem all students and training programs have to face.

University training programs will address this issue in various ways, and it is our hope that you will have the support you need to become proficient in your professional writing abilities. Unfortunately, there typically is no formal course in clinical writing at most universities, and many students have not received adequate writing practice in general. Although students may have the opportunity to write term papers, essays, or journal reviews, they have not had any practice with clinical writing until they are thrust into it once they begin clinical practicum. Even then, they are at the mercy of varied supervisors who have different ideas about the level of writing skill they should possess. This is made even more complicated because supervisors may differ in their own styles of clinical writing.

It is interesting to note that one university in Florida started a pilot course in clinical writing skills in order to address the lack of knowledge and experience of its students in speech-language pathology. It was also instructive that one of the recommendations following implementation of this pilot course was the development of a "sample report book" that students could follow. According to Middleton, Pannbacker, Vekovius, Sanders, & Pluett (1992), "Providing students with sample reports and training exercises allows more training in the recognition of good writing." So, even though writing prowess improves with practice and experience, there is obviously a need for guidelines and examples of what a professionally written document should look like. This same concept applies to professional correspondence such as letters and memoranda.

Organization

All well-written documents must be organized in such a way that makes them easy to follow. How many times have you read and reread something, only to find that you still cannot discern the meaning the writer is attempting to convey? When it comes to drafting a professional document, organization includes everything from sentence structure to word usage to placement of information within the document. Most resources you find that address organizational aspects of professional writing will include a list of "must-haves" for a professional document (Strunk & White, 2000). Many guidelines used in writing business reports include some key components that relate to the business letters, thank-you letters, transmittal letters, and referral letters discussed in this chapter. In the next section, we will provide examples of some of these documents; however, we would like to introduce the following information to you at this time, as we feel it is relevant to organization and it applies to various types of correspondence.

- The letter should be written on letterhead stationary if it is from a clinical facility.

- Every piece of professional correspondence should be dated at the top.
- There should be an inside address that includes basic information such as the name, address, and affiliation of the intended recipient of the letter.
- The letter should include a professional and respectful greeting or salutation (e.g., Dear Mrs. Johnson).
- The first paragraph of the letter typically provides some background information about the sender so that the recipient of the letter knows something about the person generating the correspondence.
- The body of the letter or memo should contain the reason the document is being written and whom it is written about. It should be broken up into logical paragraphs or subheadings, if necessary.
- There should be a summary or conclusion paragraph reiterating the purpose of the letter and thanking the recipient for her consideration in reading the document.
- Prior to the signature line there should be what is known as a *complimentary closing* (e.g., "Sincerely").
- The signature line should include the typed name of the sender, her degrees, and position. In the case of students you can refer to yourself as "student clinician," "graduate clinician," or the like.

Let us now take a look at how this organizational structure applies to the various types of communication we have mentioned. In general, there are four types of letters that you may be required to write during your clinical training: referral letters, thank-you letters, transmittal letters, and business letters. These will be explained further below:

- **Referral Letter:** This will usually accompany a diagnostic or treatment report for a client you are referring to another professional for services not within the scope of practice of the SLP. For example, we routinely refer clients to physicians, psychologists, occupational therapists, physical therapists, special educators, social workers, regular educators, and audiologists, among others. This letter describes the reason for the referral and introduces the client to the professional to whom we are referring the case. Without some explanation, the professional would be at a loss to understand the purpose of the referral.

◼ **Thank-You Letter:** This will usually be sent as a follow-up when a client has been referred to you from another professional. Expressing your appreciation for the referral will hopefully serve to maintain a positive professional relationship and may result in more referrals in the future. Thank-you letters are also appropriate when a company sends you complementary materials or someone donates toys/materials to your clinic. Such letters are also used when other professionals donate their time and expertise to consult with you on a case. It is a good policy to thank people for any contributions of time, materials, or finances.

◼ **Transmittal Letter:** This usually accompanies a diagnostic or treatment report that is being sent to a professional, client, parent, or caregiver. It is not professional to simply mail a report to someone without a letter of explanation accompanying the document. Such cover letters explain why the report is being sent.

◼ **Business Letter:** This is used when writing to a company or organization in order to request a service or materials. We also use business letters to correspond with insurance companies and businesses that provide administrative support to clinics such as office supplies, copying machines, and clerical personnel. Business letters might also be used to make other professionals aware of existing clinical programs offered by your facility or announce the establishment of new services by the clinic.

All four of the letters mentioned above require organization, a specific format, and professional communication. The letters sent by the SLP not only represent the individual practitioner, but the facility for which she works, so they must be professionally done.

An example of each type of letter is provided in the boxes.

Sample Referral Letter

May 23, 2008

Jennifer Smith, OT
Main Street Rehabilitation
Montgomery, AL

Dear Ms. Smith:

I am writing this letter in regard to Sam Jones, a 3-year-old male, who was seen at this clinic for a speech and language evaluation on April 25, 2008. Sam was referred to us by his pediatrician due to a speech and language delay. During the case history interview, Janice Jones, Sam's mother, also described several other behaviors that are causing her quite a bit of concern.

Based on results of our assessment, Sam does exhibit a language delay; however, he is also demonstrating self-stimulating behaviors such as spinning and diverted eye gaze. Mrs. Jones reports that Sam is also a very "picky" eater, and that he "does not like things touching him." Based on results of our evaluation, as well as his mother's concerns, we feel that a comprehensive occupational therapy evaluation is warranted.

I appreciate your assessment of this very interesting child and am enclosing a copy of our diagnostic report for your review. I look forward to receiving your input on this case.

Sincerely,

Embry Burrus, MCD, CCC/SLP
Associate Clinical Professor

Enclosure

Sample Thank-You Letter

May 23, 2008

Daniel Rice, M.D.
Bayview Medical Clinic
123 Main St.

Dear Dr. Rice:

Thank you for referring James Goodwin to our clinic for a speech and language evaluation. We completed our evaluation of James on April 3, 2008, and have recommended that he receive speech therapy here at our clinic for the upcoming semester.

Our findings indicate that James continues to exhibit language and pragmatic difficulties as a result of the TBI he sustained approximately one year ago. Your assessment of his social language skills was excellent, and we appreciate your insight into this matter. Once we have James's authorization, we will be happy to send you a progress report at the end of the semester. Should you have any questions, or need further information, please contact us at your convenience.

Once again, thank you for your referral.

Sincerely,

Heather Daniels, B.S.
Student Clinician

Sample Transmittal Letter

May 23, 2008

Jennifer Smith, OT
Main Street Rehabilitation
Montgomery, AL

Dear Ms. Smith:

Enclosed please find the diagnostic report for Sam Smith, a 3-year-old male, who was evaluated at this clinic on March 2, 2008. Per our phone conversation, Sam has been referred to your clinic for occupational therapy due to sensory integration disorder and decreased fine motor skills.

Should you need any further information, please contact us at (123) 456-7890. I look forward to hearing from you and collaborating with you in the treatment of this child.

Sincerely,

Student Clinician

Enclosure

Sample Business Letter

May 23, 2008

Daniel Means, President
Therapy Works, Inc.
123 Main St.
Birmingham, AL

Dear Mr. Means:

My name is Ann Smith, and I am a graduate student in speech-language pathology at Ourtown University. I am very interested in learning more about the therapy materials that you offer for children who have feeding and swallowing disorders. I am about to begin my externship at a pediatric clinic and expect to see a number of children who have been diagnosed with these disorders.

I read in your catalog that a representative from your company will come to our university and demonstrate the products and that you offer a discount if we make a purchase following the demonstration. I would appreciate any assistance you could provide in arranging this for our students.

Thank you for your time and attention to this matter. I may be reached at (123) 456-9900, or via e-mail at a.smith@ourtown.edu. I look forward to hearing from you very soon.

Sincerely,

Ann Smith, B.S.
Student in SLP
Ourtown University

Another form of written correspondence you may use is the memorandum, or "memo." The memo is standard business correspondence, and, before the advent of electronic mail, was used more often by people communicating in work settings than any other type of written correspondence. The memo is still widely used today; so often, in fact, that you will hear references made to it throughout virtually every communication medium—television, radio, and water cooler conversations when people say, "Didn't you get the memo?"

The memorandum was designed to transmit important information in a brief, concise format.

According to the *Merriam-Webster Dictionary*, the definition of memorandum is: "a usually brief communication written for interoffice circulation; a communication that contains directive, advisory or informative matter." Thus, memoranda typically are not sent outside of the office in which you are working to other facilities. The memos you will be required to write will generally serve one of three purposes: (a) transmitting information, (b) requesting information, or (c) requesting or enabling action. We will provide a couple of examples in the boxes.

Requesting or Enabling Action

MEMORANDUM

To: Beverly Jones, Office Manager
Fr: Ashley Smith, Graduate Student, SLP
Re: Confidential file
Date: 6-9-08

I am writing to inform you that I am in receipt of paperwork from the graduate school that needs to be added to my personal and confidential file. I understand that you only receive information from students at specific times. Please let me know when would be a good time for me to get this information to you. Thank you in advance for your assistance in this matter.

Transmitting Information

MEMORANDUM

To: Dr. Ron Good, Department Chair
Fr: Ashley Smith, Graduate Student, SLP
Re: Comprehensive Exams
Date: 6-9-08

I am writing in regard to the oral comprehensive exam that I missed due to a death in my family. At your convenience, I would like to meet with you in order to discuss a time to reschedule this exam. Thank you for your understanding and assistance in this matter.

What you are most likely thinking at this point is that you would probably send an e-mail in each one of these cases; and, most likely, you would be right. As a matter of fact, electronic mail has, in many cases, taken the place of the interoffice memorandum. On many campuses, e-mail is considered an "official" communication between faculty, staff, and students. Therefore, students have the responsibility of checking their e-mail daily for communications from faculty members or the university administration. It is no excuse to say that you did not read your e-mail if an assignment is given to the class via this form of communication. Often, e-mail is exchanged between facilities for the purpose of scheduling appointments or other tasks associated with clients. In making this point, we would like to add that your e-mails, when used in the same way as the previous memo examples, should be just as well written and organized. We emphasize that you resist the temptation to use "text message" speech, abbreviations, and slang. This is not professional and will communicate to whoever receives your message a lack of professionalism. Do not make the mistake of communicating something about yourself that you do not intend. It is also wise to remember that any information transmitted electronically is susceptible to eavesdropping by hackers and others, especially if you are communicating over an unsecure connection and using nonencrypted e-mail. As we mentioned in an earlier chapter, you could be violating a client's confidentiality by sending sensitive clinical information by e-mail if it is intercepted by an unintended recipient. People can also easily access another person's computer and read e-mail that is stored on that machine or simply look over a shoulder and read the screen. The bottom line is that you must be very careful transmitting client information via e-mail. This also applies to sending clinical reports as e-mail attachments.

In this next section, we would like to mention a few aspects of writing to keep in mind when you are putting together your written communication.

Format

Using an outline each time you write will ensure the correct structure or format of your document, and generally, structure is one thing that does not change, regardless of who you are writing to or about. If you think back to when you learned to write a letter in grade school, you will recall that you were given an outline that you could use each time you sat down to write: the date in the top left or right corner, followed by the person's name and address to whom you were writing, the salutation, the body of the letter, and then, at the bottom of the page, the name of the sender. This was standard "letter writing" format, and you probably committed it to memory fairly easily. Our intention is to make the process of professional writing just as easy to learn, so that once you have mastered it, you will take that skill with you into the work setting you choose.

Tone and Language

The feeling you get when reading a document is mostly related to the tone in which the writer is communicating. Tone is sometimes referred to as the "voice" or "attitude" of a piece of writing. Voice, however, may also refer to the tense you are writing in, such as passive or active. Generally, professional documents are written in the passive voice. For example, "Michael was observed to use several multiword utterances," as opposed to "Michael said four three-word sentences."

In an earlier chapter we mentioned *professional tone* as applied to writing reports. This applies to writing professional correspondence as well. If you read a letter, e-mail, or memorandum that appears to be immature, nonchalant, or informal, you may wonder about the professionalism of the writer. So the words you choose to use, as well as the structure of your document, will convey a specific tone, and you always want that tone to be professional. For example, you might say, "Michael has difficulty staying on task, which may have a negative effect on his success in therapy," as opposed to "Michael won't pay attention and wiggles in his chair." The tone of each of these sentences is very different, not only because of the voice, but also because of the words that are used; "has difficulty staying on task" sounds professional, whereas "wiggles in his chair" does not. It may be helpful to refer to the term generator we have provided to find appropriate professional terminology. As we alluded to earlier, it is important to have a good working knowledge of professional terminology, as you will use it frequently when writing clinical documents. It is also important, however, that infor-

mation is communicated in a clear, concise manner (French & Sim, 1993). In addition, you want your communication to be appropriate for the person who will be receiving it. A letter that is being sent to a parent will not always read the same as information sent to a physician or other health care professional. Your reader should not need a dictionary, medical or otherwise, or an advanced degree to understand your letter. It has been our experience that students get so caught up in using the professional jargon they have learned that they want to "show it off." Professional terminology is not written for the purpose of impressing others with your knowledge. When communicating with other professionals, it can be a way to write detailed information in an abbreviated manner, but when communicating with parents or caregivers, it is a way to describe the results of your treatment or assessment in a way that is easy to understand—the goal is clear communication of sometimes complicated ideas. In his book, *On Writing Well*, William K. Zinsser makes this point when he writes (Zinsser, 2006, p. 8):

> Perhaps the sentence is so excessively cluttered, that the reader, hacking through the verbiage, simply doesn't know what it means. Perhaps a sentence is so shoddily constructed that the reader does not know how to read it, or perhaps Sentence B is not a logical sequence to Sentence A.

Finally, you should always pay attention to the grammar and organization of professional letters and to spelling, as well. Fortunately, most word processing programs have grammar and spell-checking tools that will alert you to your linguistic missteps, but remember that these programs are not infallible as demonstrated by the anonymous poem in the box below.

Spell Checker Blues

Eye halve a spelling chequer
It came with my pea sea
It plainly marques four my revue
Miss steaks eye kin knot sea.

Eye strike a key and type a word
And weight four it two say
Weather eye am wrong oar write
It shows me strait a weigh.

As soon as a mist ache is maid
It nose bee fore two long
And eye can put the error rite
Its rarely ever wrong.

Eye have run this poem threw it
I am shore your pleased two no
Its letter perfect in it's weigh
My chequer tolled me sew.

Anon

The purpose of the present chapter has been to bring to a conscious level the notion that *any* written communication generated by the SLP puts forth an image of professionalism. The reports, letters, memoranda, and e-mails that you produce reflect not only on you as a professional, but on the facility you represent. They must be organized in the correct format, written in professional language, and free of grammatical and spelling errors. Do not hesitate to take the opportunity to carefully review the documents you generate, because once you hit the Enter button or drop that envelope in the mailbox, it is far too late for revisions.

SECTION III

Professional Verbal Communication

9 Interacting with Clients and Families

In the previous section of the present text we have discussed professional written communication in the form of diagnostic reports, treatment plans, and various forms of progress reports. Your written communications have a profound effect on how you are perceived by others and they also serve to guide your clinical work. As a student in speech-language pathology (SLP), you will be using professional written communication across various practicum settings and we hope that the general guidelines we have provided in prior chapters will serve you well. A book about professional communication, however, should discuss more than just the writing of reports. Communication takes place through several modalities and writing is only one of them. You will find that in every practicum setting, you will participate in verbal interactions with clients, family members, other professionals, and clinical supervisors. In most cases, these verbal interactions between people have an even greater impact on your clients, other professionals, and supervisors than your written reports. Verbal interactions are pivotal in the way you are perceived by others and central to how clients, families, professionals, and supervisors form an opinion about your professionalism. Do not underestimate the importance of each verbal interaction you have with others because these exchanges have a significant impact in two critical areas. First, as we stated above, verbal interactions are the primary determinant of another person's perception of you as a professional. Second, we use verbal interactions to gain information, counsel clients, provide information, and train others to participate in the treatment process. Although we could do all of these things in written communication, there would be no opportunity for exchange of information between the clinician and others. Clients and other professionals have questions that

must be answered by the clinician. In many cases, it is important to convince clients and professionals to participate in the treatment program and motivate them to perform for greater progress in therapy. Perhaps more significantly, verbal communication adds the all-important human element to clinical practice. Face-to-face verbal interactions can often be the critical variable in success or failure of a treatment effort.

SELECTED CRITICAL ELEMENTS OF PROFESSIONAL VERBAL COMMUNICATION

From examining the table of contents you already know that we will present three separate chapters on professional verbal communication. The present chapter focuses on communication with clients and families. The next two chapters will deal with communication issues related to other professionals and clinical supervisors. There are, however, some critical elements that should be infused in professional verbal communication across all of these groups. Thus, while we discuss these variables here, you should remember that they should be part of all professional verbal communication. The elements discussed below are mainly for beginning students in clinical practicum. There are many other characteristics that have been suggested over the years that contribute to effective interviewing and counseling. For example, Shipley (1997) lists the following: sensitivity, respect, empathy, objectivity, listening skills, motivation, and rapport. Many of these are subsumed under the five elements we discuss below. We have chosen only five variables because they are probably among the most important for beginning clinicians, and they relate to professional communication. Figure 9–1 illustrates five factors that should be present in all professional interactions and we will briefly discuss each of them in the following sections.

Show Respect

This component is something that should be part of any communication, whether professional or casual, but it is especially important for clinicians (Shipley, 1997). We want our clients, other professionals, and clinical supervisors to feel as if they are treated with respect for their infinite dignity and worth as human beings. Clients and families come to us for services to ameliorate a communication disorder that is having a negative impact on their lives. They may feel embarrassed and at a disadvantage when they have to come to a professional for help. We ask them for personal information about their problems, which again makes them feel vulnerable. These clients/families need to believe that the professional will treat them and the information they provide with dignity

and respect. So how do we behave when we treat clients respectfully? First of all, it is common that at the beginning of the clinical relationship we refer to clients/families with a respectful term of address such as "Mr. Jones" or "Mrs. Smith." This form of address connotes a professional relationship and communicates respect for the client/family member. Obviously, after working with a family for a period of time you become more familiar and the person may say, "Please, call me Michelle." It is then appropriate to refer to the client/family member as he or she wishes, but we believe that it should be their call. Imagine yourself in a hospital after having a stroke. You have been deprived of all dignity and are in a vulnerable position. Then a stranger comes into your room and says, "How ya doin', Charlie?" This kind of familiarity from someone you have never met is not a respectful form of address. It is much more professional to say something like, "Hello, Mr. Smith, I'm Suzanne Jones, a speech therapist. I understand you've had a stroke and are having some trouble talking." Just by using a term such as "Mr. Smith," you have communicated respect for the patient. When dealing with other pro-

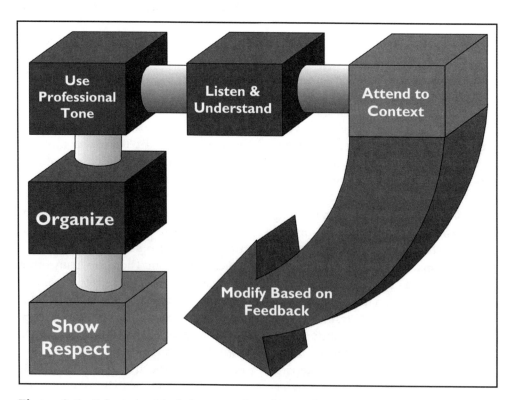

Figure 9–1. Selected critical elements of professional verbal communication.

fessionals it is always good to begin by using their title (e.g., Dr. Smith) or calling them "Mr.," "Mrs.," or "Ms." You will find yourself dealing with psychologists, physicians, teachers, physical therapists, occupational therapists, and many other professionals who are consulting on your client. When you are at a staffing or introducing other professionals to family members, referring to them more formally is a sign of respect. As everyone gets to know each other, you will know when to refer to other professionals less formally. Regarding verbal communication with supervisors, it goes without saying that you want to strike a respectful posture with someone who is evaluating your practicum performance.

Respect for a person is also communicated non-verbally and by the physical environment in which you communicate. Your nonverbal behavior should suggest that you are genuinely interested in his concerns and take the interaction very seriously. You should conduct professional communications in a comfortable, professional environment that protects client confidentiality and provides an opportunity for the person to express himself without distractions. Making a person comfortable in a professional environment shows that you respect him as an individual and care about his concerns.

Organize

You will recall from an earlier chapter that we suggested that one of the most important parts of writing diagnostic reports is organization. Having an organization to the information you provide makes the report follow a logical sequence and increases its intelligibility to the reader. It is exactly the same with professional verbal communication. No one wants to listen to a person who just rambles on in an unorganized stream of consciousness. A clinician has particular goals in mind when talking to clients/families, other professionals, or supervisors. For example, our goal might be to obtain specific kinds of information from a client or family member during a diagnostic interview. Obviously, it would help to have thought about the types of information you need and mentally prepare for the interview. Some clinicians make general notes regarding areas of discussion in the diagnostic interview. It is much better to be organ-

ized than to complete the interview and discover that you have not asked some important questions. Another example might be that you are asked to participate in a multidisciplinary staffing of your case with other professionals. Again, these other professionals do not have time to listen to a rambling, unorganized discussion of your dealings with the client. You should have your remarks outlined and any visual aids (e.g., handouts, treatment data) prepared prior to the staffing so that you can present a coherent description of your client. When talking with your clinical supervisor, it is always a good policy to organize your information prior to the meeting. If you are talking about treatment progress or you have questions for your supervisor, these can all be organized and discussed in a logical way rather than haphazardly. Thus, it is clear that verbal interactions with clients/families, other professionals, and supervisors are not mysterious and unpredictable. You should prepare for these meetings ahead of time by organizing what you will say. You might have to do this on paper in the beginning, but with more experience you will be able to mentally organize your discourse.

Use Professional Tone

You will recall that we introduced the notion of *professional tone words* in Chapter 4. By using these words, clinicians make their reports sound professional, and it is no different in verbal communication. The key in verbal interaction, however, is that the clinician must judge whether such terms would be appropriate for the person involved in the communication. For instance, if talking to a classroom teacher, a term such as *literacy* would probably be understood. Similarly, you might use the word *cognitive* when talking with a psychologist. On the other hand, if you were talking with a parent who had an eighth grade education, it would not be appropriate to use a term such as cognitive because he may not have been exposed to that word. Thus, it is important to use professional tone words in verbal communication as much as possible, but you should always consider the background of the listener. In cases where professional tone words would confuse the communication, it is important to simplify, while at the same time not sacrificing accuracy.

Listen and Understand

Professional verbal communication is a two-way street. You are not talking with clients/family members, professionals, and supervisors just to hear the sound of your own voice. Thus, it is important to be a good listener when engaging in professional verbal communication. Most counseling texts suggest that it is critical that we listen to others for both the *content* and the *affect* of what they are saying (Crowe, 1997). The notion of content refers to the actual words and information that the person is providing. For instance, if a parent says, "Jeremy said his first word at age 3," the content would be the literal information provided by the mother. However, if the mother said the above utterance while a tear ran down her cheek and her voice broke in the middle of the sentence, this illustrates the affect or emotional tone of the utterance. Attending to both the content and affect of utterances in professional verbal interactions is very important. In the above illustration, we might want to engage the mother in further conversation about how she feels about her child's disorder. She may simply need to vent her concern and disappointment, or she may need a referral to a counselor if it seems like the feelings are affecting her life negatively. The point here is that we would not want to simply jot down that her child said his first word at age 3 and ignore the clear expression of emotion. The same principle applies when dealing with other professionals. If you are trying to engage a classroom teacher to help with language stimulation for a preschool child and she says, "Sure, I'll help with the speech therapy; I don't have anything else to do," there is something more in that utterance than her willingness to assist in treatment. She is obviously feeling overwhelmed with her job and views your suggestions as an intrusion. If you attended to this emotional tone, you might indicate that you will be willing to come into the classroom and handle certain activities or assure the teacher that your suggestions can be implemented while she handles her regular routine.

The listening principle also applies to communicating with clinical supervisors. If you ask for therapy suggestions and your supervisor asks, "Have you looked in your class notes and in the library?" the real message is that you need to take more responsibility for coming up with ideas rather than being "spoon-fed" by your supervisor. Never underestimate the importance of not only *listening* but *understanding* your partners in verbal communication.

Attend to Context

Every verbal communication takes place in a context. The idea of communicative context has several components to which a professional must attend. Specifically, we are referring to (a) who you are talking to, (b) where you are talking, and (c) the feedback that you receive from your communication partner. First of all, you must consider the person to whom you are talking. This person possesses certain background knowledge, has a specific position in the social/professional hierarchy, and represents a unique cultural history. Any verbal communication must take into account these "who" variables whether you are speaking to clients/family members, other professionals, or your clinical supervisor. Let's say you are working with a Native American family from a lower socioeconomic level who has a child with a language disorder. You cannot assume that this family will inherently understand the nature, assessment, and treatment of child language disorders. Thus, your use of professional tone words will have to be reduced in favor of more "client-friendly" language. Several sources report that many cultures are not comfortable in revealing personal information to relative strangers (Battle, 1997; Roseberry-McKibbin, 1997). A good clinician will take this into account and perhaps postpone some of the more sensitive questioning until after a stronger relationship has been formed with the family. It is easy to see that appreciating the context of professional verbal communication is an important variable in dealing with clients. It is also significant when dealing with other professionals. For example, when you talk to a classroom teacher, you can assume background knowledge about the educational milieu and the types of problems typically seen in SLP and teacher collaborations. You can use "educational" vocabulary and even some vocabulary specific to SLP if you have worked with this teacher before. If this teacher is also the principal of the school, she is treated with more respect and deference than a teacher with no administrative role in the school hierarchy. If the teacher is Hispanic, you want to make certain that you do not make any cultural gaffes in your conversation that might be offensive to a member of that ethnic group. Thus, the "who" of verbal communication partially defines how the conversation takes place.

The "where" of verbal communication also dictates the nature of a professional conversation. If you are talking in a hospital setting it is appropriate to use medical terminology shared by physicians, nurses, OTs, and PTs. You can assume that a term such as *FIM score* will be understood by most people you are working with. But, even though you are in a hospital, you must also remember the "who" factor. If you are talking to a family member of a teenager with a head injury, the term FIM score will be meaningless, and you have to modify your language to suit the listener. Similarly, when talking in an educational setting, you might assume that most teachers, special educators, and school psychologists share knowledge of certain terminology unless it is very discipline specific. At any rate, it is fine to throw around terms like *IEP* and *benchmark* with most educational personnel; just don't mention *diadochokinetic rate*.

Modify Based on Feedback

In any professional conversation with clients/families, professionals, and supervisors, there will be turn-taking and interchange of both verbal and nonverbal communication. Sometimes, even if you have been respectful, organized your thoughts, used professional terminology, listened to content/affect, and attended to context, there will be miscommunication and error. This is why a professional always examines the nonverbal and verbal feedback from a conversational partner. If you are explaining the assessment results to parents and they begin to look quizzically at you, it is time to rephrase your utterance so that it can be understood. If you are explaining your test results/recommendations to a physician and he starts shaking his head, you will need to address any concerns that are present in your next utterance. Thus, it

should be no surprise that professional verbal communication forms a feedback loop by which we constantly monitor our conversation and make changes to optimize communication. Ideally, we generate the optimal utterances on the initial attempt, but in cases where there is misunderstanding, we always have an opportunity to clarify.

THE VALUE OF EXPERIENCE

As we stated earlier, the critical elements discussed above are a part of any professional verbal communication, whether it is to clients/families, professionals, or supervisors. As a beginning student in clinical practicum you have no doubt marveled at the verbal ability of your supervisors in talking with parents, family members, and other professionals. How do they get to be so confident and able to think on their feet? Well, like many other enterprises, it all gets better with experience. You will find that in the beginning of your practicum experience you will probably not be given assignments to talk with clients/family members on your own. Instead, you will probably sit in on sessions where your clinical supervisor carries out the interview or parent training or presents information at a staffing with other professionals. One reason why your opportunities at professional verbal communication will be severely limited at the beginning of practicum is that this is a skill that does not come naturally to any student. You first need to observe competent models of professional verbal communication from experienced clinicians. As you progress in clinical practicum, you will be trusted to take on more of the responsibilities of verbal communication with clients/families. By the time you are finishing graduate school, you will have seen many different styles of interaction with clients and their families. You will then find yourself incorporating the styles of various supervisors with your own personality that will ultimately result in your own style of professional verbal communication. Before you graduate, you should have had the experience of conducting a variety of types of verbal communication with little supervision as you talk to clients, families, and other professionals.

CONTEXTS OF PROFESSIONAL VERBAL COMMUNICATION WITH CLIENTS AND FAMILIES

There are at least six major contexts in which you will be using professional verbal communication with clients and families: (a) a diagnostic interview with parents of a child client; (b) a diagnostic interview with an adult client; (c) a diagnostic interview with the family of an adult client; (d) conducting training sessions for developing a home treatment program; (e) discussing treatment progress with clients/families; and (f) counseling clients/families about treatment issues. It is beyond the scope of the present text to provide detailed coverage of how to conduct interviews for every disorder seen by the SLP. Similarly, it is impossible to do justice to the field of counseling in a couple of short chapters. We refer you to other sources for a more detailed treatment of interviewing and counseling (Crowe, 1997; Emerick, 1969; Haynes & Pindzola, 2008; Shipley, 1997). We will talk generically about dealing with clients/families in the six areas mentioned above. Although there are disorder-specific considerations for every type of communication impairment, there are also some general principles that can be applied to interviewing and counseling no matter what the disorder. We will provide a brief sketch of some salient points from each area in the following sections.

Three Important Issues Common to All Diagnostic Interviews

We will be discussing some factors related to conducting diagnostic interviews with parents, family members, and adult clients in the next portions of this chapter. First, however, we should mention some important issues that are common to any diagnostic interview with any of the above groups.

The Interview Setting

Remember that one aspect of professionalism is the context in which clinical activity takes place. We want the interview room to be professional in appearance.

This means it should be neat, clean, comfortable, and private. You must consider that the parents, client, or family members will be revealing personal information that should be kept confidential. This means that we do not perform a diagnostic interview in a waiting room or hallway. There should be some privacy provided for activities such as in an office or treatment/evaluation room.

Setting the Tone

A diagnostic interview is not simply a social chat. The interview is directed by the clinician, although the parents, client, or family members may not be aware that it is a directed conversation. It is up to the clinician to set the tone for the interview by telling the parents, client, or family members what will transpire (Matarazzo & Wiens, 1972; McQuire & Lorch, 1968). The box shows a brief example.

> Mr. and Mrs. Jones, I wanted to start by saying that I'm pleased to meet both of you and your son Brad. To begin, I want to let you know what we will be doing today for Brad's evaluation. First, I know that you have filled out our case history forms and I have read those before this meeting. During the first part of our meeting today I would like to clarify several things you mentioned in the paperwork and see if I can get some more information that will help me as we do the evaluation. So, first we will talk about Brad, and then I will be giving him some tests and taking some samples of his communication. After we are all finished with the assessment, we will meet with you again and let you know our preliminary findings and recommendations. At that time you might have questions that we can answer. It's better to save your questions for later on because we will be able to answer them more fully after seeing Brad. Right now, I would like to ask you some questions about Brad because you know him better than anyone else and can give me examples of what he is having difficulty with.

Notice how the clinician speaks formally, yet in a friendly manner. Note also that the clinician has sketched out how the evaluation will flow from obtaining information and assessing the child to providing information and making recommendations.

The Presenting Story

Most authorities on clinical interviewing suggest that clients come to the experience with a "presenting story" that they have rehearsed prior to the actual meeting (Emerick, 1969). You have no doubt experienced this yourself as a patient going to a physician for diagnosis of a medical problem. On your way to the doctor you might think about the types of symptoms you have been experiencing and what you have done to help yourself. Some people even talk through this presenting story in their car while driving to the doctor's office. It is important to let the patient reveal the presenting story because it contains his reason for coming into the clinic, his perception of the problem, and any misconceptions he might have regarding the situation. There are some ways to elicit the presenting story in the box.

I'd like to begin by having you tell me what led up to your coming to the clinic for an evaluation.

So, how can we help you with Brad?

I know you've filled out our paperwork, but sometimes it is helpful to have you provide a little background in your own words about your concerns.

I'd like to start by having you tell me about your concerns and why you came in today.

Notice how the clinician leaves it open ended so that the parents can describe in detail their concerns and issues. These can be followed up by questions from the clinician when information is not clear. It is almost always good to ask parents for an example of behaviors they are concerned about. Sometimes clients, parents, or family members have misconceptions about their child's situation. We should always listen to these but not correct the client at this point in the interview. Later, when we provide information about the evaluation we can clarify any misconceptions that exist. For example, see the box.

In the diagnostic interview the mother says:

Brad mispronounces everything and people can't understand him. I've got this Uncle Calvin who is mentally retarded and nobody could understand him either. We hope that Brad isn't, you know, slow like Calvin.

After the evaluation the clinician says:

Earlier you mentioned a concern that Brad might be misarticulating because of mental retardation. First of all, most people with mental retardation who misarticulate have problems with vocabulary and sentence structure and show delays in many areas such as motor skill, social development, play, and activities of daily living. Brad has near normal language and he has normal social, motor, and self-help skills. From Brad's language ability, his play, and the way he is interested in complicated videogames, I can tell you that he does not behave like a child with mental retardation. Research has shown that most children with misarticulations similar to Brad's are of normal or above intelligence. In his case we feel the problem is confined to speech sounds.

There are three classical parts to a diagnostic interview, whether it is with parents, clients, or family members. According to Haynes and Pindzola (2008), the interview is designed to do three things *in this order*: (a) obtain information, (b) provide information, and (c) provide counseling if necessary. Let us briefly go over these three components of a diagnostic interview as illustrated with parents.

Diagnostic Interview with Parents

One of the most important objectives of a diagnostic interview is to obtain information from the client/family. It is usually wise to focus on background information first to help you compensate for omissions and ambiguities in the case history. In many instances, responses on a case history form raise more questions than they answer. For instance, the parent might have indicated that the child takes a lot of medications, but has failed to mention what specific types of drugs are taken. You would want to follow up on this by saying, "In the case history you mentioned that your son takes several medications. Can you tell us what they are?" Sometimes parents will say something very general or ambiguous that you would like a specific example of, such as, "Joey has behavior problems." There are many types of behaviors that are typical in children (e.g., tantrums) and those that are of more concern (e.g., lighting fires, abusing animals). It is always good to solicit examples from parents if they have been ambiguous. You can see that there can be many general issues to clarify in a diagnostic interview, and usually the initial part of the interview is spent disposing of these background issues. But we are not done obtaining information yet. Some writers have characterized the diagnostic interview as a "funnel" in which we begin talking about general information and then focus more tightly upon specific issues (Emerick, 1969; Stewart & Cash, 1974). Thus, we rarely go into a diagnostic evaluation of a child knowing nothing about the disorder of major concern to the family. Typically, we will have read case history forms that have been completed by the parents prior to the actual evaluation date. In most cases, the case history information will have a statement of the problem according to the parents, and this gives us a general guide to planning the evaluation. For instance, the parents might indicate that they are concerned about dysfluencies, hoarseness, language development, or articulation errors. These statements of concern help us to focus the evaluation and the questions posed in the diagnostic interview. If the problem is hoarseness, you will want to ask questions about activities that could contribute to vocal abuse/misuse. You will also want to know how the vocal quality changes throughout the day, and if it had a sudden or gradual onset. There are many areas of questioning that are specific to each disorder of communication and you should be prepared to ask them in an evaluation.

As you are selecting standardized and nonstandardized measures to use in the evaluation session, you should also be thinking about questions you would like to ask the parents when they come for the assessment. Organization has been a common thread winding through this text, and you can see that it is important in conducting a parent interview. Beginning clinicians should write down areas of concern in which more information is needed. We do not suggest writing down *specific questions* because, as mentioned in a previous section, you do not know the parent's level of understanding. You could craft a specific question, and it might be too technical for some parents or not specific enough for others. Jotting down "areas" that you want to research is a more flexible approach. So, for example, if you have a concern about hearing loss and the parent has not addressed this in the case history, you should ask about hearing in the interview. The major point here

is that you should never go into a parent interview unprepared. You should arrive at the interview with a legal pad that has specific issues written on it *in a logical sequence*. If you want to get more information on the biological foundations of communication, group your questions appropriately (e.g., hearing, motor skill, injuries, illnesses, medications). For example, do not skip from hearing to play to social friendships and then back to illnesses. Obviously, organization and planning of an interview can be done for any suspected area of concern in communication disorders whether it is language, phonology, fluency, or voice. You should look carefully at the case history information and then in your class notes and textbooks for specific background information that should be probed for the type of communication disorder of concern to the parents. Before the evaluation, it is a good idea to show your proposed interview protocol to your supervisor. We guarantee you that the supervisor will be impressed with a student who has thought about and planned a clinical interaction with parents.

We need to mention an important thing about the conduct of a diagnostic interview. The clinician is in control of this conversation and must direct it from the outset. Interviews are not the same thing as a social chat that moves randomly from topic to topic. You should set the tone for the interview by telling the family how it will proceed. You can indicate that the first part of the conversation will be to get information from the family because, after all, they are the most knowledgeable about their particular situation and concern. Once the parents know that you want information to use in your assessment, they usually cooperate by giving examples and answering your questions. Sometimes parents want to ask questions during the obtaining information portion of the interview (e.g., "What causes a child to have delayed speech?"). This is guaranteed to get you off the track of obtaining information and it is best to stick to your plan. You might say, "I'll be able to answer you better after the evaluation when I've had a chance to see how Henry does on our tests. We'll have plenty of time to go over everything, but right now I want to learn about what you have done to help him at home." Once you have all the information you require, it is time to do the actual evaluation and gather data on the child's performance on standardized and nonstandardized tasks.

After the evaluation tasks, the parents will no doubt want to hear something about the results. No one wants to come to an evaluation and be told to go home without at least some preliminary information. Obviously, you will not have time to formally score all the standardized tests and transcribe/analyze a language sample on the day of the evaluation. You will, however, know some general pieces of information about the child's performance and be familiar enough with the case to know whether or not treatment is recommended. Thus, providing information can be conceived as having three parts. The first part of providing information is to summarize as many of the test results as you can, if only on a general level. Although you may not have scored a test, you will know that he missed a lot of items on certain subtests, or that he was able to complete other items without difficulty. You will know about language errors he made from a conversational sample. From your knowledge of normal communication development, you should know whether or not the child's performance is similar to other children at this age level. After summarizing the general test results, you then move toward interpreting the test results and talking about prognosis. The parents need to know what it means when you say that he performed poorly on an articulation test, but his performance on language tests was normal. For example, parents may not know that phonological and linguistic disorders are often co-occurring, but in Henry's case, his main difficulty is with the speech sounds. They also need to know that because he was stimulable, has normal hearing, has an interested family, and has no language problems, he has a good chance to perform well in therapy. After summarizing and interpreting the test results, you are ready to make recommendations. You might recommend treatment two times per week for 30 minutes for work on specific phonemes or phonological processes. The point here is that you have provided information in a systematic way moving from test results to interpretation to recommendation. Again, organization is key to professional verbal communication. The box gives an example of providing information to parents of a child who was evaluated for a fluency disorder. Notice that the clinician summarizes the test findings, and then moves into interpretation and finally into recommendations. Note also that the clinician leaves time for the parents to ask questions.

The Results

Well, we've finished all of our testing of Michael and I'd like to tell you what we found. First of all, Michael did fine on all of the language and articulation tests we administered, so he seems to be developing sentence structure and speech sounds in a normal fashion. He also has normal hearing according to our screening. We took a large conversational speech sample and we did notice various types of dysfluency in his speech. For example, he repeated whole words, phrases, parts of words, and some individual speech sounds when he talked. We also noticed some tense pauses in his speech where he abruptly stopped talking, breathing, and voicing. Another thing he did was to put filled pauses like "uh" in his sentences when he had trouble. He also showed some struggle behavior when he seemed to get stuck on a word.

Interpretation

So the language, hearing, and articulation results are very positive and we have no concern in those areas. In the area of fluency it is important to note that most children Michael's age repeat words and sentences as part of normal development and he has those kinds of repetitions in his speech. You mentioned earlier that you were concerned about the development of stuttering. Some of the things that suggest the possible development of a stuttering problem are things like repeating parts of words such as syllables, and repeating individual sounds such as "k-k-k-k-kite." Also, tense pauses and struggle behaviors are associated with the onset of stuttering in many children. You also mentioned in our earlier interview that Michael's uncle had a stuttering problem. If we look at all these things together, we feel that Michael is not merely producing normal developmental dysfluency, but is showing some warning signs of continuing to stutter.

Recommendations and Prognosis

Because Michael is less than 4 years old we feel he has a good chance to become more fluent with therapy. Usually, the earlier a stuttering disorder is caught, the better the outlook. Also, because his language abilities are normal and his parents are concerned, he has a lot of positive things going for him. We would recommend that Michael come to therapy two times a week and that we work with you on some things that might help him be more fluent at home. Now, are there any questions you have for me?

The final component of the diagnostic interview is providing counseling, if necessary. In the vast majority of cases, no counseling issues arise in the diagnostic session. Sometimes, parents will react emotionally if they are hearing for the first time that their child really has a communication disorder. Perhaps they have been holding on to the hope that their child is really normal and just wanted to have that notion confirmed. Another issue might be concern over finances and if they can afford to pay for treatment. Most universities have sliding fee scales, or the parents can be referred to the public school system where treatment is free of charge. The point here is that if a parent expresses a real concern, emotional or not, you cannot just send him home to ruminate about it. If there is something you can say to ease the concern, you should do it. Again, in most cases this will not be necessary, but remember what we said in an earlier section about listening for content and affect in your clients.

Diagnostic Interviews with Adult Clients and Their Family Members

You will notice that we have combined the next two areas of professional verbal communication in dealing with clients and families. Mercifully, many of the same issues we raised in the previous section on diagnostic interviews with parents apply to these other groups. We are still conducting a professional interview and we still have our three goals of obtaining information and providing information and counseling, if needed. There are some slight differences in dealing with adult clients and their families. First of all, when dealing with parents, we are really not asking the young child questions during the interview. The parents are the most reliable informants for younger children. For older students, however, it is critical to involve them actively in the interview. In the case of adult clients, however, they can speak for themselves and should be allowed to do so unless they are incapacitated. For example, a patient who has had a stroke and cannot talk would not be able to provide information during the evaluation. In that case, interviewing a family member is a reasonable method of obtaining this information. We must always be careful, however, to maintain the dignity and respect of the patient. We do not want to talk about him as if he is not there. It is always good to involve the patient in the interview, if for no other reason than to confirm what the family member has said. Some clinicians ask questions first of the patient, and then turn to the family member if he is unable to respond. Then you can ask the patient if that information is correct, or make a comment related to the new information. Even if you do not ask a question, you can let the patient know where you are going with the interview. For example, you might say, "I'd like to learn a little about the work that you did with the government. Is it all right if I ask your wife to tell me about that?" Again, you are still trying to obtain information from the client or family member, just as you would do when talking to parents. In most cases, adult clients are fully capable of speaking for themselves. Adults who stutter or have minor language problems, phonological disorders, or a vocal disorder can give you information directly during the diagnostic interview. For all adult clients, you must organize your questioning in a logical sequence for the disorder area that is of concern to the client, just as we illustrated in the previous section on the parent interview. The order of the diagnostic interview, however, does not change. First you obtain information, and then you administer various diagnostic tests. After testing, you provide information about test results/interpretation and make recommendations. If the client has major questions or concerns that require brief counseling, you provide it as needed.

Conducting Training Sessions for Developing a Home Treatment Program

In most treatment approaches that seek to improve speech and language, it is desirable to develop a home program to facilitate the generalization of communication skills learned in the clinic to other environments. Usually, the success of home programs depends to a large degree on the amount of direct training provided to the family and the clinician's ability to communicate what is to be done. Therefore, for a program to be successful there must be some type of organization in presenting the information to parents or clients. In child language, for example, Paul (2001) presents many parent programs that take a structured approach to training for generalization to the home environment. In other words, for a home program to succeed, the parents or family members must be specifically trained to carry out the generalization activities. You are not establishing a home program when you walk the client down the hall after therapy and suggest they do a little of this and a little of that. Such suggestions, although not harmful, are not likely to be implemented correctly or implemented at all, for that matter. On the other hand, if you use the last 10 minutes of your treatment session to invite the parent or family member into the therapy room and actually show him what to do and let him try it, that is a different story. This gives you the opportunity to critique the way he is performing the technique and provide reinforcement and suggestions. Our point here is that home programs can enhance generalization, but home programs are not as effective without specific training. This training is done through the use of professional verbal communication.

The first step in training a parent or family member is to organize your training regime. There is that word again: organization. You must put some thought into what you want to train, the procedure to be used in training, and the most effective way to communicate this to the parent or family member. This is applicable to any type of training whether it is directed at language stimulation, reduction of vocal abuse, reacting to dysfluency, or generalizing gains made in correct production of misarticulated phonemes. One important thing should be clear from the outset. We want the home program to involve fairly simple, straightforward, and doable tasks that can be easily fit into the daily routine. The parent should not be trained to do complex treatment tasks that are difficult to learn and carry out reliably. The general progression of such training has several components, no matter what the disorder area targeted. First, the clinician must tell the parent/family member about the general goals of the home program. If it is a child language case, it might be the use of recasting at home to facilitate generalization.

Specifically, let's talk about a child who substitutes him/he and her/she. This child might say, "Her is my sister." We are working on the correct use of pronouns in clinical sessions, but we want to involve the parents in a home program to facilitate generalization. Much research has shown that recasting has been effective in training language across many different groups of children and a variety of language structures (Nelson, Camarata, Welsh, & Butkovsky, 1996). So, in this first step, we need to tell the parents that there is research that supports the use of recasting in language training and this is a technique that is fairly easy to learn and implement during daily interactions in the home environment. The clinician might define recasting as restating the child's incorrect utterance in a correct manner. For example, if the child says, "Her is my sister," the parent should say, "Yes, she is your sister." Recasts can easily be woven into conversations and they do not require the child to imitate or correct the utterance. All they do is immediately give the child a correct model of a sentence that he has produced incorrectly.

After outlining the technique that you want the parents to use, you move on to step two. In the second step of parent training, you actually demonstrate the technique with the child in the therapy room with the parent watching. In this way, the parent can see the procedure in action and it is not simply an abstraction that was talked about in step one. After several demonstrations, you move on to step three. In the third step, the parent is encouraged to try the technique with the child and the clinician provides feedback about effective use of the technique and anything that might be changed to make it more productive. In the fourth step, the parent is asked about situations in the home environment where recasting might be used. For instance, the parent might say that a lot of conversations with the child occur in the car when running errands and going to various sports practice events. This is a good time to have conversation and use recasts. Finally, the parent is asked to make some mental notes about the child's correct production of the target language structure. That is, we want the parent to notice if the child is beginning to use the correct forms more often.

It is clear that training parents/family members to do any type of home program is done by professional verbal communication. We explain, model, monitor, and charge the parent/family member with the responsibility of implementing the technique. This applies to everything from articulation disorders to vocal abuse to stuttering. The key is that the training is organized and professionally done by the clinician.

Discussing Treatment Progress with Clients and Families

It is the responsibility of any competent clinician to provide feedback to clients and/or families about how they are making progress in treatment. Ideally, this is done by presenting behavioral data showing that performance has changed over time. Again, this is done by professional verbal communication. Certainly, you can give copies of treatment reports to clients/family members, but in most cases such reports are written in terms that are more appropriate for SLPs and other professionals. It is always a good policy to sit down with clients/family members and take stock of progress or lack thereof. In the university clinic, for example, the end of the semester is a good time to have such a conference.

As in any professional verbal communication, organization is again a central issue. You should not sit down with clients/family members to casually discuss clinical progress without adequate preparation. Some obvious components of that preparation would be the data gathered throughout the semester, and in most cases it is good to display the data on a chart or graph. If the graph shows an increase in performance of treatment targets or a decrease in errors, most parents are satisfied that they are getting their money's worth. When explaining treatment progress, it is a good idea to recap the goals targeted in therapy and how they relate to the data presented. Another part of a treatment progress conference is to talk about the next set of goals that will be targeted in the next semester and ask for feedback from the parent or client. Although we all would like to make progress in treatment, there are cases in which the conference will demonstrate a decided lack of progress. If the graph is not moving away from baseline levels, then the discussion with the parents might focus on variables that need to be changed in order for progress to occur. For instance, a child who comes to treatment once a week for 30 minutes and is not making progress might need to try coming twice a week in order to have a positive response. Again, the data you present will support your suggestion. Do not forget in these progress conferences to solicit client/family member feedback. Are there things they are especially pleased with regarding the treatment? Are

there aspects of the therapy they do not understand? Do they have any concerns or issues they would like to raise? All of this is done using professional verbal communication and it is a critical component of a good clinical relationship with clients or families.

Counseling Clients and Families about Treatment Issues

On a realistic level, counseling in a clinical relationship is designed to solve problems and/or deal with feelings related to the treatment regime. Many types of problems may be associated with treatment such as irregular attendance to therapy sessions, lack of progress, unrealistic expectations on the part of the client/family, feelings of hostility or discouragement related to the treatment, lack of motivation, explaining changes in the treatment approach, transition to another service provider, or referral to a professional from a related discipline (e.g., psychology). Actually, the issues listed above might very well account for most of the counseling efforts in treatment encountered by students in clinical practicum, but there are certainly others we have not raised. As a student, you probably will not be entrusted with more sensitive issues that require counseling; this will be left to your supervisor. Counseling typically requires more of a long-term relationship with a client. It takes time to build trust and demonstrate clinical competence. You may only be seeing a client for a single semester, whereas your supervisor may have been involved with the case for a longer period of time. You will, however, have to deal with the day-to-day occurrences that happen in any therapeutic relationship. Thus, it is the goal of this section to provide a *general* view of the process of communicating about counseling issues rather than an all-encompassing set of guidelines. For more detailed coverage of counseling we direct you to other sources (Crowe, 1997; Shipley, 1997).

Figure 9-2 shows a very basic process of identifying and dealing with treatment issues using professional verbal communication. This is fundamentally "problem solving"; however, you will see that confronting problems in clinical work often leads to talking about feelings and perceptions that are more sensitive than a simple social conversation. We would

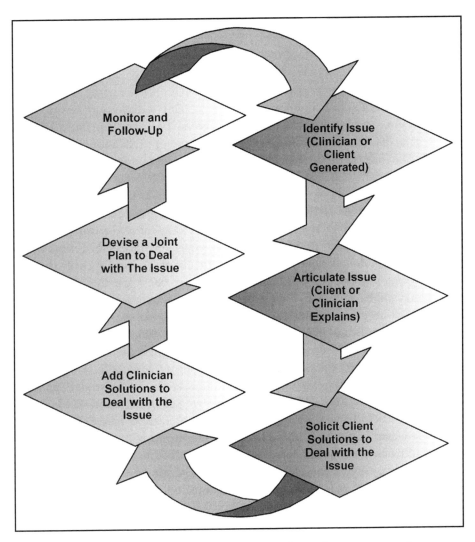

Figure 9–2. Counseling with clients/family members about treatment issues.

like to be clear at the outset: Counseling a client is serious business that takes years of training and experience to perform well. Just to give you some insight, Crowe (1997) discusses some of the following counseling opportunities that arise in SLP, depending on the client's age and type of disorder: (a) feelings of anxiety, grief, guilt, isolation, and anger; (b) denial of the problem; (c) dealing with a guarded prognosis; (d) self-concept; (e) cultural barriers; and (f) inaccurate perceptions and nonproductive attitudes. Shipley (1997) raises the specter of clients who are paranoid, overprotective, talk too much, are depressed, and may even contemplate suicide due to the changes in their lives after a stroke, laryngectomy,

or degenerative neurological disease. Obviously, we do not expect students in training to delve into the psyches of their clients and deal with these major emotional and life issues. In some cases, even the experienced SLP must refer such seriously involved clients to professional counselors or psychotherapists. Most of the time we can deal with clients having a bad day by just being human, listening to them, and demonstrating that we understand their feelings. No one who is feeling depressed wants another person to deny the validity of his feelings and pretend that everything is all sweetness and light. Clients who become frustrated and depressed about their abilities after a stroke might say, "I used to be able to do woodworking in my workshop, but since the stroke, I can't use my tools. That was my favorite hobby and now I can't do it." A validation of their concern would be an appropriate response, such as, "I know how much you loved woodworking and it must be very frustrating not to be able to do that anymore." Remember the content and affect concept. In most cases, for practicum students, there are more basic issues to deal with that involve professional verbal communication. If serious counseling issues come up, the student needs to (a) recognize the issue, (b) address it if it is a fairly simple and straightforward problem, and (c) alert the clinical supervisor if the problem seems beyond his ability to deal with. It is always better to err on the side of caution rather than dabble in issues you are not equipped to handle. Your own experience will be a guide as well. For example, once you have counseled parents on children's behavior problems with the help of your supervisor, you should feel some confidence in addressing similar issues with a new case. On the other hand, if your client with a laryngectomy says she has no friends and does not want to live, you probably need to get some help from your supervisor. Thus, the approach we are taking to counseling is a series of steps for addressing problems that arise with clients in your practicum experience. We will briefly discuss each step below, and guess what? Organization is a major factor in counseling, just as in every other aspect of professional verbal and written communication.

The first step in counseling about treatment issues is to identify the problem. In some cases, the client/family member will be the person who identifies an issue of concern. For example, after a treatment session one day, a client might express dissatisfaction with the amount of progress being made in therapy. Your first reaction might be to act defensive about such a comment and you might feel bad about your performance as a clinician. A positive aspect of this comment is that the client has brought it out into the open and has not internalized it and simply sabotaged the treatment by not trying or failing to attend therapy sessions. A good clinician simply cannot let this comment go by and not deal with it. Thus, we have a situation in which a client has identified an issue (dissatisfaction with treatment progress) and the clinician must find a way to explore the problem and suggest solutions. The second step

in this process is to obtain the client's perception of the problem. Typically, the clinician can act as a facilitator to gain more insight into the issue. For instance, the clinician might say, "Let's talk about this for a while. Tell me some specific things that you are not satisfied with in our treatment approach or your progress. Then we can make some adjustments to the therapy or talk about your progress and how we can improve our approach." This opens up a "can of worms," but you can clearly see that allowing a client to go through the motions in treatment sessions while harboring such feelings is not productive. In some cases, there is simply a misunderstanding of the goals or unrealistic expectations on the part of the client. These can easily be dealt with by counseling the client on the difficulty of treatment and providing examples of the range of progress made by many clients working on the same type of communication disorder.

Sometimes there is a very specific issue that is bothering the client. For example, a client who stutters might be frustrated with clinical exercises involving easy onset and slowed speech rate because no generalization to daily situations is seen where the stuttering still occurs. Again, this can be dealt with by further explanation of the techniques, or more realistic situations can be integrated into the treatment in which the techniques can be used to facilitate fluency in everyday communication. Whatever the situation, it is always better to address it than ignore it.

After identifying the issue and articulating it, the focus should be on potential solutions to the problem. If you have not learned this already as part of your life, solutions are generally better when arrived at jointly by the people experiencing the problem. It is a wise clinician who solicits client solutions to a problem and then suggests some additional solutions to the mix. So we ask the client, "What do you think we can do to make better progress?" In some cases the client may say that more treatment sessions are needed. In other cases, the client may feel the clinician is not being aggressive enough in treatment. Other cases may want some different aspects added to the treatment approach. The next step is for the clinician to add possible solutions to those that the client has provided. Be sure to reinforce the client's suggestions if they are reasonable. "I really like your suggestion of using more realistic situations in therapy. Actually, I've got a whole file of real-life activities that we can arrange in order of difficulty and start using next week if you like."

So both the client and clinician have made positive suggestions for the treatment approach and the next step is to agree on a joint plan of action. If the client likes some of the ideas that were generated in joint discussion, the plan needs to be formalized. "Okay, it sounds like we are in agreement about the problem and some potential things to try in order to solve it. I'll bring my list of activities on Monday and we can prioritize them so we can work toward you being able to use your techniques in more realistic situations." Now, it might occur to you that the client may not be ready to produce fluent speech in more difficult situations. What if the person fails at the new activities? This is not all bad, because it may just be the dose of reality the client needed to justify more work on easy onset and slower rate in the clinic. All the counseling in the world may not make the client feel good about boring clinical activities, but experiencing difficulty on higher level tasks might bring home the realization that a bit more practice on the easy onset and slower rate is not such a dreadful idea after all. If the client is successful at more difficult tasks, it merely shows what a good clinician you are because you have responded to client suggestions that allowed faster treatment progress. If the client is not successful, again you have been responsive to concerns, but you were correct in your initial judgment of client abilities, and it is now clear why you started at that level.

The final step in the process is to monitor how the plan has worked. After trying out the plan agreed upon by the client and clinician, it is always a good idea to take stock of how things are going. "Well, we've tried some more realistic activities and you seem to be responding well according to our data on your dysfluencies. How do you feel about your progress in therapy now?" This gives you an opportunity to attain closure on a problem that has been solved, and it also opens the door to making adjustment in the treatment that will fine-tune the approach.

Remember that we said the counseling issue might be raised by either the client or the clinician. For instance, the clinician may be concerned about the client's attendance, the inconsistent use of practice outside the clinic, or the lack of motivation. Any of these issues can and should be raised if they are on the clinician's mind. "We have you scheduled for therapy three times a week, and yet you are only coming one or two times. I'm afraid that this might be having an impact on your progress. There are a lot of reasons why people come inconsistently ranging from scheduling to money to transportation to motivation. So, tell me about why you are having trouble getting here and maybe we can come up with a plan to make things better." Again, you could just let it slide and not say anything, but you are not dealing with the underlying problem. Opening the door to discussing such issues is much better than ignoring them and hypothesizing all sorts of reasons that may not be true. Whoever raises the issue, client or clinician, the important thing is that the concern receives your attention. These concerns are dealt with exclusively by professional verbal communication as you identify issues, articulate them, solicit joint solutions, devise a cooperative plan, and monitor the plan to determine if it was or was not successful.

The purpose of this chapter was to illustrate some basic principles of professional verbal communication with clients and families. As a student in clinical practicum, you will do far more communicating verbally than on paper with your clients and family members. This verbal communication is a platform by which you obtain information, provide information, and deal with problems that arise in the course of your clinical relationship. Always remember to be respectful, organized, professional in your language, a good listener, and attend to the context of communication so that your utterances will be appropriate in terms of the environment and the client's knowledge base and culture. If you remember these things when communicating verbally you will be perceived as a professional. Also, know that problems are bound to arise in any clinical relationship. It is always best to deal with such issues earlier rather than later. Whether the client raises the issue or you must bring up a sensitive problem, these concerns can be dealt with in a systematic way using professional verbal communication. The problem must be identified and discussed. A joint plan of action must be devised using input from both clinician and client. Finally, a mechanism to monitor whether or not the problem has been solved must be put into place. Such problem solving is always a challenge, but it is a natural part of clinical responsibility, interaction, and ultimately success.

10 Interacting with Other Professionals

In the beginning of your clinical practicum experience you will probably have little opportunity to directly interact with other professionals. This is because initial practicum assignments are typically in the university clinic. Usually such clinics are staffed solely by speech-language pathologists and audiologists, unless the clinic operates in tandem with other departments on campus such as special education, psychology, or health professions. Although such models exist on university campuses, they are not the norm. As you progress in your practicum experience, you will find yourself interacting with more professionals from other disciplines as you are assigned to rehabilitation centers, hospitals, schools, or long-term care facilities. Even in the beginning, however, you might have the opportunity to collaborate with other professionals on a case you are working with in the university clinic. For example, you may be working with a child who has a language/phonological disorder. It is possible that this child is attending public school and is also receiving treatment from the school SLP. This child will also have a classroom teacher and may be receiving other services from a specialist in learning disabilities. Thus, even though your work is confined to the university clinic you might come in contact with these other professionals for a variety of reasons. First, you might be interested to know about the IEP goals that your client is working on in the public schools. To find this out, you have to contact the school SLP either in person, by telephone, by e-mail, or by letter to obtain the relevant information. A second reason to contact the public school professionals is to determine how your approach at the university could make the best contribution to the child's overall treatment regimen by coordinating your goals with those of the school personnel. For instance, they might be working on literacy issues and grammar but have little time to work on phonology and pragmatics. The university program could coordinate work on a variety of goals so that some are not ignored or duplicated across settings. This coordination takes professional verbal communication. A third reason to contact the school professionals is to determine how the work you are doing with the child in the university clinic is generalizing to the school environment. You may want to visit the school and observe your client's communication in the academic setting. During this visit, you will no doubt come in contact with professionals who work in the school system. A final reason to contact the school personnel is to determine what curricular materials might be used in your therapy to result in maximum generalization. Most authorities in school-age language disorders suggest that treatment activities incorporate some curricular material such as vocabulary and discussion topics so that the child can receive an academic payoff in addition to the communicative gains.

Depending on the type of case, there may be other professionals dealing with your client simultaneously. Some campuses, for instance, have programs for children with autism. In such programs, the child may be seen in a preschool program in the department of special education or psychology and you might be doing your treatment either in the university clinic or in these other departments. Either way, you are in a position to interact with other professionals. Thus, you can see that interaction with other professionals can take place even when you are operating in the sheltered environment of the university clinic. As we said above, such interactions will only increase as your practicum experiences take you to other settings throughout graduate school.

In Chapter 9 we outlined several critical elements that should be part of professional verbal communication with clients and families. These elements were showing respect, organization, use of a professional tone, listening/understanding, and attending to the communicative context. All of these elements, crucial to interacting with clients/families, are just as important when dealing with other professionals. We gave several examples of how these factors apply to our conversations with professionals in Chapter 9. We just wanted to bring them back to a conscious level for the present chapter. It is assumed that you will attend to these critical elements of interaction in all your communications with professionals from other disciplines.

CONTEXTS OF VERBAL COMMUNICATION WITH OTHER PROFESSIONALS

There are at least four contexts in which you will be likely to interact with professionals from other disciplines: (a) consultations, (b) staffings/meetings, (c) collaboration, and (d) solving problems in informal daily interactions. We will discuss each of these below to give you a flavor for how they unfold.

Consultations

In most instances the purpose of a consultation is to access additional information or a different perspective on your client. There are several reasons why the SLP will consult another professional about a case. In the first instance, you might want to consult a professional to obtain information that will assist you in your treatment program. We mentioned above a situation in which you might want to obtain information about the school curriculum and/or goals that the school SLP is targeting in treatment. In most cases, to be done effectively, this necessitates a face-to-face meeting. It is difficult to cover all the information over the telephone or in written communication, the latter of which does not allow for questions and clarification. A second reason to consult another professional is to ask for help that is discipline specific. For instance, in working with a child who has autism

you might have questions about how to deal with behavior problems that occur in treatment. In your search for answers you might ask a person from the psychology department to consult on the case. During this consultation, you could meet with the psychologist to discuss your concerns either in the psychology department or in the speech and hearing clinic. You might want to ask the psychologist to observe the child and provide suggestions on dealing with behavioral issues. As you progress in practicum to other work settings, it is not unusual to ask other professionals such as physical therapists, occupational therapists, nurses, or physicians for a formal or informal consult on a patient you are working with. Remember, there is a difference between an informal consultation and a formal referral for an evaluation by another professional. Informal consultations are usually a professional courtesy given to one person by another. Formal referrals for evaluation are done on a fee basis and often need doctor's orders or other administrative paperwork to occur. It is one thing to refer a child for a psychological evaluation, and quite another to ask for "input" from a colleague who works in your organization. As mentioned in Chapter 3, it is crucial to obtain a signed release of information from the client/parent before involving another professional in order to protect client confidentiality. Never underestimate the importance of obtaining a release of information before *any* consultation is done. Assuming we have permission, we might find the SLP asking the occupational therapist or physical therapist about positioning issues when working with a client who has motoric disorders. Because these other professionals are working with the client on activities of daily living, they are usually more than happy to give suggestions about positioning the client for activities involving the SLP. Similarly, other professionals will ask the SLP about the communicative status of a patient with whom they are both working and how best to have successful interactions. Such informal consults are part of working together as a rehabilitation team.

When asking another professional for a consultation, it is important to remember that you are requesting a favor. Thus, you can see why showing respect, organizing your request, talking professionally, listening carefully, and attending to context are critical. The box illustrates an example with a psychologist:

Telephone Contact

Hello Dr. Jarvis, this is Madyline Smith and I'm a speech-language pathology student working in the university speech and hearing clinic. My clinical supervisor suggested that I contact you about a child I'm working with on language development. The child has autism and is exhibiting some behaviors that we are having difficulty dealing with. I was wondering if it would be possible to set up a short meeting with you to get your input on what I might do to make my treatment more effective?

The Meeting

Thank you so much for taking the time to talk with me about Kevin. I would greatly appreciate any insight you might provide in this case. So I don't take up too much of your time, I've brought along some video examples of the behaviors I am having trouble with, so if you look at my camcorder screen you can see what I'm talking about. I'm especially concerned when Kevin hits and spits during therapy like in these examples. Right now, I'm dealing with this by telling him "No" when he does these behaviors, but it doesn't seem to reduce their occurrence. Do you have any suggestions?

Initial Contact in the Hallway

Hi, Mrs. Johnson, I was wondering if I could get some advice on Lester Hollis. Because you are his teacher and know how he responds, I'd like your input on combining some classroom material into his language goals. If you are willing, I'd be happy to come to your classroom after school some day for a few minutes to get your opinion on what I'm doing to incorporate the curriculum into his therapy.

The Meeting

Thank you so much for meeting with me about Lester. I've brought the materials I'm using with him and I wanted to show you how we are trying to incorporate American government into our language goals. You can see that I've made up an organizational chart we can use when we discuss how the government works to make laws. I was wondering if there are any other important government processes Lester and I can discuss in therapy that would also help him in the classroom.

Notice how the clinician called to set up the appointment to see if the psychologist was willing to consult. Also, note that the clinician got right to the point, showed the psychologist what she had concerns about, and indicated her current approach in dealing with the behavior. You can see that organization was important in obtaining this consultation. There was preparation time in terms of looking up the correct telephone number, making an appointment, selecting video examples of the behavior that was of concern, and telling the psychologist how the behaviors are currently being handled. After the meeting, it should go without saying that the clinician thanks the psychologist for the consult. It is always a nice touch to give feedback to the other professional, especially if her suggestion has been implemented and it was effective. Everyone likes to hear that her advice was followed and helped the situation. Also, it never hurts to let the other professional know that "if there is ever anything we can do for you on a case in the future please let us know." The box gives an example in a school system of consulting with a teacher:

Notice how the clinician approaches the teacher in a respectful manner and makes a convenient time to talk about the student. At the meeting, the clinician is well prepared and organized and asks specific questions about how to apply classroom work to treatment.

Consultation is an important component of the relationship between various disciplines. As your career progresses, you should be prepared to both request consultation from and provide consultation to other professionals. Verbal communication is the major vehicle for consultation, and for success to occur, it must be done in a professional manner.

Staffings and Meetings

In many work settings there is often the opportunity to "staff" a case that has common interest to a variety of professionals. Staffings usually focus on pulling together multidisciplinary assessment information from a variety of professionals, or they concern progress reports on a client who has been in treatment for a period of time. The two environments where staffings are most common are medical facilities and school systems. In some university clinics, students are asked to meet for the purpose of discussing their cases as part of a "grand rounds" experience or merely a case presentation. Such experiences in the university clinic give the beginning student a chance to organize and cogently present information on a client to faculty and peers in the training program. Presumably, it prepares these students for presentations they might have to make in other work settings later in their practicum experience. For example, in school systems there are IEP meetings and other opportunities to discuss the progress of students receiving therapy. In medical facilities, staffings are common and are attended by representatives of all health professions involved with the patient. Often, these staffings are weekly, especially in facilities where the patient is staying for a limited time frame.

The conduct of a staffing is much like any meeting where there is an agenda. The purpose of the staffing is for all of the professionals who work with the patient to update the team regarding progress toward goals and any difficulties that may have arisen since the last meeting. Typically, one professional (and it could be from any discipline) directs the meeting. For example, in dealing with children, this person is often called the *case manager* and will facilitate the conduct of a staffing in which a child's treatment progress is discussed by the educational team. In some facilities the staffing concerns many patients, each of whom must be talked about by all relevant professionals. In these types of staffings, time is of the essence and each professional is allotted only a few minutes to report on the patient's progress. Thus, you will only have a short period of time to let the other professionals know how a particular patient is progressing toward goals. This is one reason why FIM scores are commonly used in medical facilities. It does not take long to report that "Mr. Jones has moved from a level X to a level Y on language comprehension." In other settings, however, the meeting or staffing concerns only a single client. For instance, there are clinics that provide in-depth multidisciplinary evaluations, and the purpose of the staffing is for each professional to provide detailed information on her assessment and finally to engage in a discussion of the combined results to arrive at treatment recommendations. Obviously, in this type of meeting you will have the floor for a longer period of time and go into significantly more detail. In some medical settings, difficult and complicated

cases are staffed in detail with lengthy presentations by different professionals and a group discussion of recommendations.

If you are scheduled to participate in a staffing of your client next week, there are several things you should do in preparation. First of all, you should find out the nature of the staffing in terms of time allotted to each participant. It makes a great deal of difference if you have to prepare a 5-minute presentation or a 30-minute case summary. For our purposes, let's assume that you are scheduled to talk for 15 minutes about your case and the progress he has made in treatment over the last 3 months. If you have read this textbook thus far, you already know that merely showing up at the staffing with no preparation is not an option. Organization and preparation give you the opportunity to make a successful and informative presentation. Lack of preparation will result in a poor to mediocre presentation that will not reflect positively on you or the facility you represent.

After finding out the type of meeting you will be attending, you should assemble all of your data on the client so you can determine the information that will be the most relevant. In this particular case, you are charged with presenting information on the client's progress over a 3-month period. Thus, you probably will want to spend most of your presentation time on this topic rather than an extensive reiteration of the client's case history or his status 6 months ago. Although it is certainly acceptable to mention some historical information and intake data, your focus should be on the past 3 months. In many cases the same professionals sitting around the table will have attended a meeting on this same client 3 months ago when you talked about earlier therapy progress. In this case, they are familiar with background information and how the client first responded when entering the facility. So how do you prepare yourself to present the treatment progress over the last 3 months? A logical place to start is to mention all of the goals you were working on during that period. This can be followed by the presentation of treatment data on each goal, perhaps supported by graphs or handouts. The final portion of your presentation might focus on eliminating goals that have been accomplished and the establishment of new goals to be targeted in the next 3 months. Notice that the presentation is organized, focused, and packaged to fit into the time allotted. It is also important to remember that you must take into account your audience when you are presenting information at a staffing. Although you can use professional terms that cross disciplines, any concepts unique to SLP should be explained in easy to understand language to avoid confusion.

If you are not the first one to present, it is often useful to refer to the presentations of others to validate points you need to make in your summary. For example, if the occupational therapist reports that the patient has difficulty paying attention while learning self-help tasks, you might say, "Just as OT indicated, I have also noticed attentional difficulties during my language treatment tasks." It not only shows that you are listening, but it validates the observation of someone else on the team and helps to consolidate information on the patient.

Staffings are not just serial reports by representatives of varied disciplines. Subsequent to individual reports, there is usually discussion centered on trying to integrate the reports and modify future goals based on client progress. Often, the discussion turns to problem solving in difficult cases. An important thing to remember is that you are part of a team that must reach some sort of consensus. You must strike a balance between raising issues and solutions you feel are important and allowing others to do the same. Staffings in which professionals provide no input and those in which a person dominates the group are equally unproductive. Remember, the client is the most important consideration in any staffing.

Staffings are an important part of working as a SLP. They should never be taken lightly because you are not only representing yourself and your facility, but the entire profession of speech-language pathology as well. Staffings are accomplished almost exclusively with verbal communication among professionals, so students should take advantage of the opportunity to watch supervisors and graduate students perform in this arena.

Collaboration

For years, SLPs have cooperated with professionals from other disciplines in what has become known as a *consultative model* or *collaborative model* of treatment. In these models, professionals from varied disciplines work together to facilitate treatment progress in a particular client. Haynes, Moran, and Pindzola (2006) outline collaborative models in terms of interdisciplinary, multidisciplinary, and transdisciplinary approaches to therapy. Each of these approaches involves members of various disciplines, but the interaction among the professions is quite different. In multidisciplinary approaches, for example, each profession sees the client separately and there is very little cross-disciplinary planning. There are separate and discipline-specific evaluations, goals, treatments, billing, and parent/family conferences. As mentioned above, a staffing may occur at some point, but it is usually discipline specific. A multidisciplinary staffing would consist of each discipline presenting what it did for the client and the progress achieved on targeted goals.

Interdisciplinary approaches are usually a bit more collaborative in that various professionals might, at least informally, discuss the client and try to cooperate on goals. There are still separate treatment sessions for each discipline, but perhaps the biggest difference between multi- and interdisciplinary cooperation is that there is a bit more joint goal-setting and communication among the professionals.

In transdisciplinary collaboration there is the most communication and cooperation among professionals. The psychologist may actually work on communication goals at the same time as behavioral objectives. The SLP might incorporate motor skills into the treatment sessions for communication goals. The classroom teacher might assist in communication goals in the context of the classroom. There is a large literature on consultative models used in assessment and treatment and it is beyond the scope of the present text to elaborate on this research (Damico, 1987; Ferguson, 1991; Frassinelli, Superior, & Meyers, 1983; Fujiki & Brinton, 1984; Magnotta, 1991; Marvin, 1987; Montgomery, 1992; Moore-Brown, 1991).

It is important, however, for beginning practicum students to see that, depending on where you are doing therapy, you may experience a variety of types of treatment approaches. Each of these different models of treatment involves changes in the types of professional verbal interactions you will have with other disciplines. These range from very little communication and collaboration (multidisciplinary) to frequent and close communication and collaboration (transdisciplinary). You should be able to see at this point that in multidisciplinary approaches you are pretty much on your own in terms of assessing, developing goals, providing treatment, and evaluating treatment progress. On the other hand, in a transdisciplinary model you will have to communicate and cooperate with all the other disciplines involved to assess, develop goals, provide treatment, and evaluate treatment outcomes. In such a model you might be doing your therapy in the classroom environment instead of a therapy room. You may also be reinforcing academic goals in your therapy and behavioral goals suggested by the psychologist. In transdisciplinary models, everything is negotiated among the professionals involved, and this is all done by means of verbal communication. Some guidelines for conducting collaboration with other professionals were presented by Haynes et al., 2006). We will briefly paraphrase some of those points below:

Administrative matters:

■ When using a collaborative model, it should not be an informal process, but should be formalized at a meeting. The group of professionals should assemble and discuss the collaborative treatment approach for the client.

■ After the discussion, someone on the team should be designated to write down the treatment approach and everyone's responsibilities so that it can be included in the client's folder.

Attitudinal variables:

■ You should listen attentively to other professionals on the team and "show respect and consideration for the other team members' expertise, questions, opinions, decisions, concerns, or goals involving the client" (Haynes et al., 2006, p. 33).

■ You should assume a positive attitude and be sure to reinforce other professionals for their good ideas.

■ Make sure you have studied the client's folder and have some issues/concerns that you want to address to the group.

Conducting meetings:

■ Make sure that each professional has an opportunity to provide input.

■ Use "situational leadership" in which the professional with the most expertise on an issue (e.g., psychologist, SLP, teacher, PT, OT) takes the lead in discussing the topic.

■ It is important for team members not to come to the meeting with a preconceived idea of what will be done. This is not working on a team; it is assuming that you have the best idea and it should be implemented. These meetings are not designed for one person to convince the other professionals to approach the treatment according to a single perspective or plan. The group should discuss the tactics for dealing with the problem and devise a joint approach to accomplishing goals.

■ Do not use too much discipline-specific jargon. This interferes with communication and is a subtle way of putting other team members in a subservient position of having to ask for clarification.

■ The team should devise specific goals for the client, assign responsibilities for targeting them, and discuss how they will be evaluated and who will assess the progress toward the goals.

■ As mentioned above, this should be formalized in a report following the meeting and included in the client's folder.

No doubt, you can see that collaborating with other disciplines takes time, planning, preparation, and professional verbal communication.

Solving Problems in Informal Daily Interactions

In any relationship, including professional ones, there is always the possibility that interpersonal difficulties can arise. Although there are many areas in which interpersonal problems can occur, in our experience there are three major categories likely to be encountered by beginning students in clinical practicum: (a) mistakes, (b) misunderstanding/miscommunication, and (c) crossing discipline boundaries.

Making Mistakes

The first area of interpersonal difficulty involves making errors or mistakes in assessment, treatment, or clinical reporting. First of all, *everyone* makes mistakes at some point. You tend to make fewer mistakes with experience, so students in training are a "high-risk" population. Hopefully, your clinical supervisor can help you head off major errors, but there are always some that slip through. One thing is for certain: once you make an error you should learn from that experience and not let it happen again. That is one difference between you and your clinical supervisor: The supervisor has had the opportunity to make errors over a long period of time and learn from those mistakes, and you are only beginning. What kinds of mistakes are we talking about? Obviously, you will make many mistakes in writing clinical reports, but those are between you and your supervisor. Those errors never make it out into the world for others to see. In verbal communication, however, you do not have the luxury of a rough draft and soliciting comments from your supervisor. Thus, those verbal errors are not as easily retrievable. For example, you might have given information at a staffing that was incorrect or misinterpreted. In this case, the other professionals on the team may not know that the scores you presented were wrong and take them at face value. Obviously, if you said the child scored in the 80th percentile on a language test, but it was really the 8th percentile, this represents a major discrepancy. In cases like this, it is important for you to admit your mistake as soon as possible and explain the true nature of the situation. Everyone makes mistakes; it is only when you do not acknowledge them or try to hide them that you get into trouble. Other professionals will respect you more for finding and admitting your error than if you did not report it at all. Imagine your embarrassment, if after working with the client for a long time some other professional finds a discrepancy and brings it to the attention of the group at the next staffing.

The same principle applies to treatment objectives. Let's say you recommended in a staffing that certain goals should be a priority for language intervention. After working with the client for a while, you realize that the goals you set were far too ambitious and difficult for the client and you need to select other goals that are more realistic. Other professionals will respect your clinical decision to change your goals after considering the client's performance.

Because we know that students in training are mistake-prone, there are several proactive principles to keep in mind. First, you should check and double-check your work so that mistakes can be found and corrected before you communicate them verbally. You cannot do a good job of professional verbal communication if you are relying on inaccurate data. A second principle to keep in mind is to think about what you are planning to say before you open your mouth. Make sure it is based on accurate data and not speculation. Make sure you think about saying it as professionally as possible. If you are not sure, ask someone such as a mentor or supervisor who is willing to provide helpful advice. Remember, once you say something, it is out there in the environment. You cannot, as they say, "unring a bell."

Misunderstandings and Miscommunications

Another area of potential difficulty with other professionals is misunderstanding and miscommunication. This is not just limited to the use of technical, discipline-specific language; it can come at you from many directions. The box shows you some examples.

OT: Mr. Smith's family told me that you said he will not ever be able to feed himself. Feeding is one of our major goals and I don't appreciate you telling the family he won't be able to do it.

(Actually, you only said to the family that Mr. Smith was having some difficulty with feeding himself, among other aspects of activities of daily living, including communication. You never said anything about prognosis or the future. This was a misunderstanding and exaggeration by the family that was passed on to the OT).

Teacher: Bobby's parents told me at our conference last week that you said I wasn't doing a very good job of teaching him how to read. I don't like it when other people undermine what I'm trying to do in the classroom.

(Actually, you said to the parents that children with language impairment often have difficulty learning to read and might need some extra help from time to time. The parents interpreted this as the teacher not doing her job.)

SLP: Johnny seems to be missing many of the cognitive attainments that are associated with language development.

Psychologist: SLPs are not qualified to assess intelligence; that is the job of the psychologist!

(Actually, you were only talking about certain cognitive play behaviors such as object permanence, means-end, symbolic play, and functional use of objects that are related to language development. You were not making judgments about his overall intelligence.

School Principal: My teachers tell me that you are complaining about the room that you use for speech therapy. You need to know that we have space limitations here and everyone cannot have exactly the type of room they want.

(Actually, you did say to two teachers that because you were assigned to work in the cafeteria on the stage behind the curtain, it was a bit noisy for some of the distractible students, especially when the custodial and kitchen staff were setting up for lunchtime.)

All of these situations were the product of misinterpretation or miscommunication among various professionals. In each of the instances the result was one professional being upset because of something someone thought you had said or done. These situations are unavoidable due to human nature. People do not always render an accurate report of what others have said, and the result is misunderstanding. If these situations are not dealt with, it could result in damaging the professional relationship you have with people from other disciplines. As a result, it could lead to unsuccessful collaborations and ultimately hurt the clients we are trying to serve.

In all of these situations, the antidote is effective professional verbal communication. First, it is important to notice the fact that a person is upset over something she feels you have done. This may be communicated directly as in the above examples, or indirectly by nonverbal cues or reports from others. Again, it is important to look at both content and affect of what someone says to you. Once you perceive there might be a problem, you need to confront it as soon as possible. Negative feelings incubate and typically grow worse without bringing them out into the open. So you need to communicate to the other person that you understand what she is feeling.

In the first example in the above box, you might say something like, "That kind of statement is very upsetting to me, and I know it must be to you as well. I know that you are working on feeding, and if the family wants to know about prognosis, they need to talk to you. Let me see if I can clarify what happened. The family was expressing some frustration about how little progress he was making. I recall telling the family that Mr. Smith had difficulty in many areas including communication, movement, feeding, and cognitive issues and that it is a challenge to have so many things to work on at the same time. I don't know how they translated that into a negative prognosis for feeding, but I'm sorry for the misunderstanding. I would never make statements to a family about something in your field. You are the expert on those issues, and I value our working relationship." Notice several things. First, the response validates the person's feelings about being upset. Second, the response tries to address the concern directly and put it in the context of what actually occurred. Finally, the tone of the response gave respect to the other professional's expertise and role in dealing with feeding issues. It might have been easy for the OT to just ignore the comments from the family, but if that happened, resentment could build for the SLP and a relationship could be impaired. It is always good to confront such issues head on. If there is a logical explanation or misunderstanding, most people will accept this as a resolution to their concern. If, on the other hand, you have made a mistake or a misstatement or have actually said an unprofessional remark, you need to apologize for it and move on. It is easy to misspeak or to make a statement in confidence to someone you trust, only to have it revealed at a later time. Optimally, it is a good policy to never say anything that you do not want another person to hear. Then, all you have to worry about is misinterpretations, but at least you won't have to apologize.

A final area of possible communication difficulty with other professionals revolves around crossing discipline boundaries. Professionals are known to exhibit a certain amount of "turfism," meaning that they perceive specific areas and procedures to be part of their field and no other's. If another professional "steps on their turf" they become defensive and upset. Because communication sciences and disorders overlap with many other disciplines, it is not unusual for us to inadvertently step over a line or two as we deal with other professionals. Think about it. We deal with teachers, nurses, physicians, psychologists, administrators, OTs, PTs, social workers, and other SLPs. Many of the issues we confront are the same as those dealt with by other professions. Take behavior problems as an example. Any professional that deals with a child who exhibits behavior disturbances must deal with these issues at the same time she is trying to accomplish the goals in her field of expertise. Thus, the teacher must deal with behavior during the teaching of science. The psychologist must deal with behaviors while teaching the student how to cope with them. The SLP deals with behaviors while teaching language and pragmatics to the student. At a staffing, it would be easy for the SLP to describe "the best way" to deal with behavior problems, but you can see that this risks stepping on the boundaries of the psychologist. Diplomacy is very important in professional verbal communication. It is better to say, "I'm not the authority on how to best deal with these behaviors, but here is what I have been doing in language therapy. I would be inter-

ested to get some input from Mr. Jones (psychologist) on this issue." In this example, you admit that behavior problems must be dealt with in your treatment sessions, but you also defer to the psychologist in terms of soliciting suggestions from the person who may be more qualified in behavior disturbance. In many work settings, disturbances in professional relationships can often be traced back to one person stepping on another's turf. Be wary of this next time you are tempted to give advice on topics that are only ancillary to your area of expertise.

This chapter has focused on professional verbal communication with people from other disciplines. There are many pitfalls in professional relationships, and although verbal communication is often the cause of interpersonal difficulties, it is also the solution. Keep the channels of communication open, and you will be on your way to becoming a competent and qualified professional.

11 Interacting with Supervisors

Communication takes many forms in our field including written, electronic, group discussion, and individual conversation. The importance of one-on-one conversation in our field cannot be overemphasized. We do it with colleagues, supervisors, clients, other professionals, parents, and family members. Part of professional communication is learning how to address these various constituencies in conversational interactions. In some cases we have these conversations just as a social interchange. At other times, the conversation has a distinct goal such as persuasion, motivation, justification, or counseling. In the previous two chapters we discussed professional verbal communication with clients/families and with professionals from other disciplines. We addressed some of the problems that arise and how professional verbal communication can be used to resolve them. The present chapter deals with verbal communication that takes place between supervisors and student clinicians. As you will learn during your training, the first clinical supervisors you will encounter are in the university speech and hearing clinic. As you progress in your program you will no doubt be sent off campus to schools, hospitals, rehabilitation centers, community clinics, private practices, and long-term care facilities. In each of these work settings you will be under the direction of a clinical supervisor. As we mentioned in Chapter 2, there are distinct differences between the university clinic and these other settings. The communication issues and student mistakes mentioned in this chapter can occur in any practicum setting, so we remind students to be proactive and maintain an open line of professional communication with your supervisors. Although the information generally applies to all practicum settings, we want to remind you that once you leave the university clinic, everything moves faster. You will be

seeing more clients, the schedule will be more hectic, the paperwork deadlines are shorter, and there is less tolerance for practicum student mistakes. These differences are, in large part, due to the fact that you are now working in a facility or school system where professional service delivery is expected and demanded. In the university clinic, everyone knows that it is a training program and the therapy is conducted by students under supervision. In a hospital, school, or rehabilitation facility, most of the service providers are certified professionals and students are in the minority. Also, your supervisor will not have 20 different practicum students on whom to focus. Therefore, it is possible that you will receive increased supervisory attention as compared to your experiences at the university clinic.

Interestingly, practicum students often report two different scenarios in off-campus settings. The first situation involves a more intensive supervisor-student relationship. This is the product of (a) more clients seen by the same student and supervisor and (b) fewer students to deal with on the part of the supervisor. The result is more time together talking about cases. Because the supervisor only has one or two students to supervise, more time can be spent scrutinizing your behavior. The second scenario reported by students at off-campus sites is less time available for supervisory conferencing. Because the supervisor is busy seeing clients and going to meetings, there is less time for supervisory conferences and, thus, less direction for the student. Some students liken this to being thrown into a swimming pool and told, "Now, learn to swim!" They report less time for the supervisor to explain and model techniques and elaborate on the required paperwork.

Either of the above scenarios can be disconcerting to a practicum student, but take our word for it, the student does learn in either one. In off-campus clinical environments you will no doubt feel more stress than you did in the sheltered environment of the university clinic, and this stress leads to unique problems between supervisors and students. But we are getting ahead of our story. First, we will spend some time talking about the nature of the relationship between a practicum student and a clinical supervisor.

THE EVOLUTION OF STUDENT AND SUPERVISOR RELATIONSHIP THROUGH THE PRACTICUM EXPERIENCE

Whether you know it or not, training programs are designed in such a way as to generate particular expectations on the part of students and supervisors. These expectations change in a predictable way as the student progresses through practicum. Anderson (1988) suggested a continuum of supervision showing that supervision is adapted to the situation and needs of the supervisee. As participation by the student increases, the degree of involvement by the supervisor decreases. The aim, of course, is to develop independent clinicians who are capable of self-supervision. Our own version of this relationship is shown in Figure 11-1, which depicts this change as the lesson of the linking triangles. The triangle on the left with the dotted outline represents the clinical supervisor. The triangle on the right with the solid line stands for the student. The height of each triangle represents the amount of clinical responsibility allocated to supervisor and student as time marches on in the training program. So you can see that the supervisor has a lot of clinical responsibility at the beginning of your undergraduate program as indicated by the height of the arrow indicating clinical responsibility. Note that as time goes on, the supervisor's triangle starts to narrow in terms of clinical responsibility. At the end of your graduate program, the supervisor's triangle has come to a point and indicates almost no clinical responsibility. Now look at the student triangle. The student starts the training program with very little clinical responsibility as shown by the pointed end of the triangle. As the students make their way through the program, the student triangle begins to broaden until at the end of graduate school the student is taking most of the

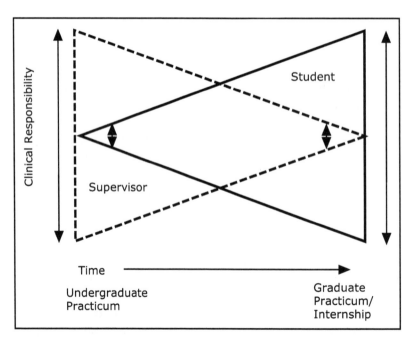

Figure 11–1. How clinical responsibility changes over time in a training program.

clinical responsibility. The triangles of the supervisor and student are exactly opposite of one another as time goes by.

This phenomenon of student practicum experience suggests that you change as you progress through your training. As a beginning student you know little practical application of your classroom materials, and with experience you become more adept at planning, executing, and reporting clinical activities. This is a natural progression for students as they become more professional and competent. The lesson here is that you should not expect to be the same in your clinical abilities at the end of your graduate program as you were as a beginning practicum student. The transformation of a student from novice to competent clinician also holds a lesson for clinical supervisors. It is axiomatic that supervisors have a sliding scale of expectations when dealing with students in training. For instance, a supervisor has much lower expectations of a beginning undergraduate student as compared to a last semester graduate student. It is only logical that expectations and grading criteria change over time in a training program. Thus, if you continue to behave as a beginning undergraduate student in terms of taking clinical responsibility, your clinical practicum grade will suffer as time goes by. The expectation is that you will profit from your classroom work and practicum experiences to become more self-reliant and take more clinical responsibility for your cases.

Sometimes a source of difficulty between students and supervisors is a mismatch of expectations between the two individuals. For example, your supervisor may be expecting you to take more clinical responsibility as you approach your third semester in practicum, and you might still feel the need for more help and direction by your supervisor. This mismatch can result in frustration for both parties and a lower grade in practicum for the student. Remember, during your clinical evolution the expectations of supervisors steadily increase based on your past practicum experience. You will know when such a mismatch in expectations occurs when supervisors ask you to independently plan, ask you for rationales, and ask you to research your classroom notes for hints on how to handle your client. Another symptom of the mismatch is when a supervisor laments having to "spoon-feed" you as a practicum student. This is your cue to actively take more clinical responsibility and come to planning sessions with your own ideas instead of waiting to be directed by your supervisor.

THE SUPERVISORY RELATIONSHIP

The relationship between the practicum student, clinical supervisor, and client is a unique blend of service delivery, clinical teaching, and student learning. Although the major goal must be the clinical progress and welfare of the client, this is also used as a teaching-learning experience between supervisor and student. In an ideal relationship, the client makes optimal progress, the supervisor can accomplish teaching goals for the student, and the student learns the targeted clinical skills. Sometimes it works exactly this way, but other times there is an imbalance. You can well imagine that this is a very difficult balancing act. The supervisor is not simply doing therapy by proxy using the student as a delivery system. The student is not a neutral conduit through which the supervisor dispenses treatment to the client. True, the student delivers the therapy and learns the critical skills of listening, motivating, taking data, and interpersonal communication abilities with clients. But the student training goal goes beyond the face-to-face skills that occur in the treatment room. In supervisory conferences, the practicum student must learn to understand *why* the treatment goals were selected, how they were arranged in the appropriate sequence, and the proper way to conduct tasks with the client.

Even after all of this preparation, an unavoidable part of clinical practicum is that the student will still make errors in judgment and behavior. Making mistakes and problem solving how to correct them is a valuable part of the learning process. If the goal of a university clinic or practicum setting was simply to do the best therapy for the client, the supervisor would provide the treatment. Clearly, in a practicum experience, there are treatment goals that benefit the client and teaching-learning goals that benefit the student. Obviously, student mistakes can have a negative effect on client progress, so the supervisor must do something to compensate for this. In most cases, the supervisor helps to insure that the student attacks the client's problem with the very best plan possible. Supervisors do not have the luxury of letting students come up with plans that are not optimal for the client merely to further the cause of student learning. Thus, the supervisor helps the student to generate a sound therapeutic procedure and to understand how and why that procedure was developed. This is done in a supervisory conference through professional verbal communication. Another way that the supervisor levels the playing field for the client is to physically supervise many of the treatment sessions or demonstrate specific therapy techniques to insure that the student is carrying out the plan optimally. Typically, less experienced students are supervised more intensively than more experienced students. Although ASHA demands that sessions are supervised a minimum of 25% of the time, most supervisors provide as much oversight as needed, depending on the capabilities of the student and the complexity of the client's disorder.

Goals of Supervisors and Students

The ASHA Committee on Supervision (1985) discussed a number of tasks that supervisors might be expected to perform during practicum experiences with students. Hegde and Davis (1995) explain each of these tasks in more detail, and students are referred to this source for a succinct summary. We will only list the tasks expected to be performed by supervisors and students to provide you with an overview. Most of the tasks are relatively self-explanatory. First, we can expect clinical supervisors to perform the following:

- Communicate effectively with practicum students.
- Provide guidelines related to practicum requirements.
- Provide the student with ongoing feedback regarding clinical performance.
- Provide assistance in planning assessment/ treatment goals.
- Assist the student in developing competent assessment and treatment strategies.
- Provide demonstrations of clinical skills.
- Provide descriptions of record-keeping requirements.

- Encourage the student to solve problems independently and develop self-analysis skills.
- Provide assistance in developing professional written and verbal communication skills.
- Direct the student to current assessment/ treatment sources in the literature.
- Provide an objective evaluation of the student's practicum performance.
- Act as a resource, mentor, and advocate for the student clinician.

Similarly, Hegde and Davis (1995) discuss a number of expectations that a supervisor might have of practicum students. Practicum students should demonstrate the following:

- Compliance with the Code of Ethics of the American Speech-Language-Hearing Association.
- Knowledge of ASHA's preferred practice patterns and scope of practice.
- Knowledge of and conformity to the clinic's policies and procedures.
- Ensuring client confidentiality.
- Appreciating the cultural and personal background of the client.
- Evidence planning and preparation for every treatment or assessment session.
- Knowledge of appropriate diagnostic and treatment methods in terms of test instruments and therapy approaches.
- Demonstration of an ability to develop appropriate goals for assessment and treatment sessions.
- Demonstration of the ability to be punctual with both written assignments and supervisory conferences.
- Maintaining accurate and appropriate clinical records.
- Showing the ability to apply coursework information to the client and engaging in appropriate library research when existing information is not available from classes.
- Demonstrating the ability to ask appropriate questions of the supervisor in order to use this mentor as a clinical resource.
- Exhibiting the ability to engage in self-evaluation of clinical skills.

■ Demonstration of punctual and regular attendance to assessment/treatment sessions.

■ Showing the ability to accurately maintain records of clinical clock hours and information for certification forms such as Knowledge and Skill Assessment (KASA) documents.

■ Demonstration of the ability to act, talk, and write in a professional manner.

■ Maintaining open lines of communication with the clinical supervisor and reporting any concerns or significant events in a timely manner.

It is easy to see that the goals of supervisors and students overlap significantly. For instance, the supervisor wants to show the student how to develop effective assessment/treatment strategies, and this is one of the student's goals as well. From reading the above bullet points you can see that the relationship between supervisor and practicum student is no mystery. We are well aware of the supervisory goals and the learning objectives of the student. However, sometimes putting the teaching and learning goals together creates some difficulties.

CRITICAL DIFFERENCES BETWEEN STUDENTS AND SUPERVISORS

Clinical supervisors and practicum students typically differ in at least three important ways. Some of these differences can cause misperceptions or miscommunications and make the accomplishment of the above-mentioned supervisor and student goals more difficult. Let us compare for a moment the clinical supervisor and practicum student:

1. **Credentials, Experience, and Perspective:** The supervisor is usually older than most practicum students and may represent the world view of a more mature individual. Additionally, with age comes attainment of advanced degrees, certification, and licensure. Being a bit older than the student also has allowed for the accumulation of years of clinical and supervision experience. Clearly, the supervisor is "coming from" quite a different perspective than a beginning practicum student, just based on age, training, and experience. In the case of the student, he has little professional experience and fewer degrees and has only begun to embark on career training. There is a large gulf between these individuals that can be difficult to span without mutual respect and effort and professional verbal communication.

2. **Workload:** The supervisor in the university setting is responsible for a caseload of perhaps 20 to 30 clients, and this probably means 20 different students to supervise. Each of these students has a different level of classroom training and clinical experience, so each supervisory conference must be "recalibrated" to account for these variables. An early undergraduate clinician, on the other hand, may have only one or two cases to focus upon. Think of the difference between the supervisor and student just in terms of the caseload size with its attendant differences in clients, student capabilities, different personalities, disparate goals, and varying schedules. It is no wonder that supervisors have a hectic schedule as they move between observation rooms to supervisory conferences to doing paperwork. In many cases these clinical faculty manage to find time to do research and professional projects as well. It is probably true that the clinical supervisor has a much more complicated schedule than the student even when you count the student's class time.

3. **Teacher-Student Relationship:** Sometimes students beginning practicum forget that the clinical supervisor is as much a teacher as a professor who stands in front of a classroom. There are some practical differences that reinforce this misconception. First, clinical supervision is usually done on an individual teacher-student basis and there is no classroom full of students. Second, we usually meet one-on-one in an office instead of a classroom. Third, because of these individual meetings between supervisor and student there is more of an opportunity to get to know each other as people, unlike the anonymity of the classroom. We raise these differences because they often lead to misconceptions on the part of students beginning the practicum experience. The first misconception is that the practicum

does not involve the relationship between a student and a teacher. However, the practicum relationship *is* a teaching-learning experience just like the classroom, except it is highly individualized and very intensive. In a supervisory conference, there is no way to avoid answering a question like you can in the classroom. There is no way to disguise the fact that you are unprepared. Because you cannot hide, you might feel that you can get by on your personal magnetism and scintillating personality. Some students and supervisors may not want to acknowledge the real nature of this relationship and thus cultivate a "friendly" style of interacting. But, no matter how friendly you become with your clinical supervisor, the relationship is always one between a teacher and a student.

Unfortunately, there is always a somewhat adversarial component to a relationship in which one person is in a position to evaluate the performance of another and assign a grade at the end of the semester. The supervisor has the goal of teaching clinical and professional skills, and you the student should have the objective of learning them. Ultimately, the supervisor will have to make judgments about your clinical abilities, professionalism, and how you are progressing toward independence in your practicum experiences. These judgments must be made no matter how cordial the relationship between supervisor and student. Thus, it is a good policy to make your interactions as pleasant and friendly as possible, but at the same time, you must make meaningful and professional contributions to the teaching-learning relationship. Another common mistake made by students is that they sometimes think that there is no homework involved in clinical practicum because it is not a class per se. Again, this idea is a misconception that could lead the student to lower grades and a less than optimal learning experience. Practicum students are expected to "bring something to the table" from their coursework and prior clinical experiences. The supervisor will expect you to go back to your class notes and look up information relevant to your case. Sometimes you will be expected to read articles and book chapters to prepare for clinical work. Obviously, there is a lot of outside work involved in devising clinical materials, keeping track of client data, and writing goals and objectives.

The three areas discussed above can lead to miscommunication on the part of both supervisors and students. Professional verbal communication is necessary to resolve these difficulties.

REMEMBER THE PRINCIPLES OF PROFESSIONAL VERBAL COMMUNICATION

As in professional verbal communication with clients, families, and other professionals, it is important to remember the critical variables of showing respect, being organized, using professional terms, listening and understanding, and paying attention to communicative context. All of these attributes are crucial in dealing with your supervisors. You obviously want to show *respect* for your clinical supervisor because he is experienced, certified, licensed, and in the position of providing you with feedback as well as a grade. *Organization* is important when dealing with supervisors. Typically, there is only a limited amount of time available for a supervisory conference. You should prepare for these conferences just as you prepare for classes or treatment sessions. For example, you might have specific questions for your supervisor and these should be organized in a logical manner. You should also make sure that the questions you ask cannot be answered by examining your class notes or querying some other source. Your supervisor will be using *professional terminology* in conferences and you should be prepared to do the same. Finally, you must *attend to the communicative context.* When you have a conversation with your supervisor you should attend to content and affect, just as we suggested in communicating with clients or other professionals. Your supervisor might communicate frustration by using intonation, body language, or facial expression rather than words. For instance, your supervisor might say, "Didn't you cover this information in your articulation disorders class?" This could mean that the supervisor wishes you had read your class notes on a particular treatment approach so it would not have to be explained to you in a conference. One of the present authors remembers a student who had a very behaviorally-oriented supervisor. The story goes that the student arrived for a supervisory conference without her treatment data from the previous week. The student said, "Oops, I forgot my data." The supervisor replied, "Well, without the treatment data we do not have much to discuss except our opinions, do we? So this conference is over." What is the supervisor's message here? Just the literal translation of the supervisor's words that the conference was terminated? Hardly. The unspoken message was clearly received. That clinician reportedly never came to another supervisory conference without her data for the next 2 years, no matter who was supervising. Do not forget the critical components of professional verbal communication.

COMMUNICATION ISSUES YOU MAY OR MAY NOT ENCOUNTER

When we ask our students about the things that "stress them out" while taking practicum, there is a cluster of complaints that are recycled semester after semester. Interestingly, communication or miscommunication is at the root of most complaints; and all of these issues can be resolved, or at least made more palatable, by acting professionally and using professional verbal communication. Here are some of the most common issues:

1. **Your supervisor wants you to do things that were not addressed in your coursework:** All students enrolled in practicum experiences will develop a relationship with a clinical supervisor. In most cases, this relationship will be a positive one; however, there may be a mismatch between information learned in academic coursework and the goals/activities that the supervisor recommends. Such a mismatch is guaranteed to make the student feel vulnerable, incompetent, and under stress. For instance, the supervisor might recommend assessment or treatment activities that go beyond what was covered in the academic coursework, and the student has to do extra work to learn about this new approach. An example might be that the clinical faculty member has gone to a recent workshop and learned about a technique that applies to the case that you have been assigned. In this scenario you must read articles and handouts that may not be familiar to you from your academic coursework. One way to look at this is that you have been given a chance to learn about a new technique and try to reconcile it with your existing knowledge. Although the extra effort might cause stress in the short term, it is a great opportunity to learn a new treatment approach and actually try it out on a real case.

2. **Your supervisor does not allow you to do things that you learned in coursework:** Academic faculty members will sometimes report that students complain that their supervisor will not let them use techniques or approaches learned in coursework. In most cases, this is due to lack of communication between the academic and clinical faculty, and not a supervisor forbidding the use of a particular approach. When the complaining student is queried, "Did you ask your supervisor if you could add phonological awareness goals to the therapy?" the student most often replies in the negative. Most supervisors would be elated if a student suggested an addition to the treatment regimen that was based on research covered in the classroom. Thus, in most cases it is not the supervisor's fault, but the timidity of the student in suggesting additions to the treatment plan. There is nothing wrong with asking to use a technique or strategy with your client you learned in the classroom. If it is appropriate, the supervisor will probably go along with it, and if it is not appropriate it provides an opportunity for discussion as to why it should not be used with this particular client. Either way, it is a good learning experience. But you will never know without communicating your concern to your supervisor.

3. **You only have your undergraduate training and are assigned a complicated case:** In most instances, this probably will not happen. Very complicated cases should not be given to a beginning student who has not had the coursework to back up clinical planning. If, however, you are given a complex case, you should expect that

supervision will be more intensive. Remember, we said earlier that the main goal of clinical practicum is that the client make progress and not be placed at a disadvantage. No one wants this to happen. If you have a challenging case, be sure to do your part in terms of asking a lot of questions, requesting frequent feedback, and researching issues yourself in addition to the information provided by your supervisor. Again, you must speak up and tell the supervisor that you do not yet feel comfortable with planning the treatment for such a difficult case because you have never had the opportunity before. On the other hand, if you are a graduate student who has worked with many such cases in the past, you have to remember the intersecting triangles in Figure 11–1. In other words, you are expected to know a lot about dealing with cases you are more familiar with. Also, you have acquired basic clinical skills such as professionalism, problem solving, and researching the literature, which you can apply to any case, regardless of the disorder.

4. **Inadequate supervision:** The American Speech-Language-Hearing Association requires that practicum experiences be supervised according to specific guidelines. For instance, assessments must be supervised in such a way that your supervisor watches 50% of your evaluation. In treatment, the requirement is 25% observation time. These, of course, are minimums, and many cases could easily benefit from 100% supervision if the case is complex and the student clinician is inexperienced. Some students report that they would like more supervision than they are receiving on a particular case and it frustrates them that their supervisor is not more involved. Certainly, most people would want the most supervision that they possibly could get, but you have to consider workload considerations and the ASHA guidelines. Adequate supervision may not be enough from your perspective, but if it meets ASHA guidelines and your supervisor is comfortable with it, that is the end of the story. Over years of working in university clinics we have seen many supervisors. Some supervise intensively and exceed ASHA guidelines. A *very few* are the subject of student complaints. For example, some students might say, "She's never around," or "I know she wasn't in the observation room at all this week," or "We only had 10 minutes for our supervisory conference and most of the time she talked about her dog." We are here to tell you that such instances are unacceptable for clinical supervisors and most do their job superbly. If, however, you are not satisfied with the amount or type of supervision you are given, the first step is to bring this up with the supervisor. Lay out your concerns in an organized and respectful fashion. For example, you might say, "I'm concerned that I have not gotten any written or verbal feedback on my performance for the past 3 weeks. We also have missed three supervisory conferences. I know you are busy, but I would appreciate your input so I can learn to be a better clinician." If no change occurs, it is important that you use whatever channels are available in your department to communicate this concern to the clinical director or department chairperson.

5. **Oppressive supervision:** In some cases, the supervisor is so involved in the treatment that the student has difficulty feeling "ownership" of the client. For example, a supervisor may frequently burst into the treatment room and "take over" the activity. Some of this behavior is beneficial under the goal of modeling good clinical skills, and you should be grateful for the opportunity to observe. If, however, it happens too much and on activities that you already feel comfortable with, then you should voice this concern to your supervisor. Another example of a supervisor who is being too aggressive is when you are not able to participate in the goal setting for your client. When your supervisor tells you the goals, prescribes specific activities, outlines how you will keep track of treatment data, and does not allow an opportunity for student input, the learning experience is affected. Earlier, we stated that the student should have the opportunity to engage in problem solving, develop strategies for selecting goals, provide rationales, and have a role in planning. If the supervisor is telling you everything to do, it is essentially the supervisor doing therapy by proxy through the student. This is not an optimal learning experience. The student should be able to request a discussion of the treatment program and let the

supervisor provide feedback about the student's ability to plan and execute the program.

6. **Personality conflicts with supervisor:** At its very base, the relationship between a supervisor and a practicum student is an interaction between two people. Although we stated earlier that it is the relationship between a teacher and a student, this does not exclude the fact that two individuals are interacting. Just as a student can have negative feelings toward a classroom teacher or a roommate, it is possible that in the more intensive relationship between the student and supervisor negative feelings can emerge as well. This is generally no one's fault, but just the inescapable reaction of two people who rub each other the wrong way. It can be very idiosyncratic and unfair. There is little to be done about this complaint because neither the student nor the supervisor is going to change his personality. So the most productive way to think about this is that you will have scores of supervisors, bosses, coordinators, teachers, and administrators who will be overseeing your work during your career. Although most of these people will be easy to get along with, there will always be a few who are not a perfect fit. Our best advice is to be philosophical about it and treat it as a learning experience. Getting along with difficult people is a skill that will come in handy for your entire career, whether they are bosses, clients or coworkers. Try to minimize your contact time, avoid pushing any hot buttons, and be respectful of the person. As long as you perform your obligations as a student clinician in a professional and timely manner, you are doing what is required of a supervisee.

7. **Differing criteria for clinical writing among supervisors:** A major complaint of students is that various clinical supervisors have different criteria for writing reports. A student can write a report for one supervisor and receive compliments on report-writing ability. When those same phrases are used in a report for a different supervisor, they are deleted with a red pencil and the student is told the writing is unprofessional. It is true that supervisors have idiosyncratic views of how reports should be written. Although they agree on issues such as format and the use of professional terminology, there will always be unique aspects to what they prefer. The worst thing a student can do is to say, "I wrote it this way for Ms. Smith and she said it was correct." You have to decide, as the old country and western song says, "when to hold 'em and when to fold 'em." Arguing about inconsistencies among supervisors is almost always a losing strategy. The best thing to do is to find out from other students and the clinical records how a particular supervisor has approved writing in the past, and stick with that particular style. After you learn the idiosyncrasies of all your supervisors you can shift appropriately, and you have had the opportunity to learn many styles of writing. When you graduate, you can develop your own style, which will no doubt be an amalgamation of all your former clinical supervisors with your individual preferences.

7. **Differing criteria for grading among supervisors:** Just as classroom teachers differ in their grading methods, so do clinical supervisors. Students are aware that in some classes, most of the students earn As and Bs. On the other hand, there are classes where As and Bs are rare and there is a preponderance of average or lower grades. It is similar in the grading of clinical practicum, although we would suspect based on our conversations with other university programs that grade inflation is especially prevalent in clinical practicum. Most students assume that they will earn an A or B in clinic, but a C is regarded almost as an F is viewed in classroom courses. We are not certain why this occurs in many programs, but it does. Nonetheless, even within the population of clinical supervisors, there are different grading styles; some are simply harder graders than others. In order to better understand the clinical grading system for an individual supervisor you can see that it is extremely important to discuss the variables you will be graded on at the outset of the semester. Do not be shy about asking what separates an A student in clinic from one who earns a B or a C. Focus on specific behaviors so that you can put your efforts into earning the grade that you desire. Also, do not underestimate the value of frequent conferences with the supervisor to ask for specific feedback on your performance in terms of a

grade. Do not be afraid to ask, "If you had to give me a grade at this point, what would it be?" Also, query your supervisor about specific behaviors you need to change to attain a higher grade. Again, professional verbal communication is critical to resolving this issue.

9. **Supervisory conferences that run over time:** It is easy to lose track of time during supervisory conferences. Sometimes the student asks more questions than usual, or the supervisor needs extra time to explain a clinical technique that will be used in the next therapy session. Whatever the cause of running over the allocated time, this should be avoided if at all possible. Due to schedules, the supervisor has meetings, other cases to watch, or other students with whom to meet. Students have classes that abut with the supervisory conference and running over in the conference will make the student late for class. This is one reason why we recommended earlier that students become very organized about their questions and issues to raise in the conference setting. Supervisors, too, should be able to use the allocated time efficiently and not run over. If the problem becomes chronic, the supervisor will terminate the conference at the appropriate time and ask the student to become more organized. If the supervisor tends to keep the student late, the student needs to say, "I'm sorry, but I have a class this hour and I don't want to be late."

MISTAKES STUDENTS MAKE

1. **Complaining to other students:** One thing students have a tendency to do is voice their frustrations to other students in order to gain empathy and support. In most cases, this merely serves to escalate the frustration and spread it to other students. You can be certain that all you will get from your peers is support, sympathy, and validation of your complaint. The student says, "Ms. Paxton wants me to read *two articles* just to work with my client!" The other students say, "Wow, I can't believe she is doing that to you; we have so much to read for our classes. I'm glad I don't have her this semester." And so

it escalates until the whole practicum student population is walking around with stifled outrage. Complaining just for the sake of complaining does not solve anything. Actually, when the supervisor assigned the readings, it should have been clear to the student why they were necessary. If it was not clear, then the student should ask the supervisor what points in particular should be attended to in the articles and how they will be integrated into the treatment. If you understand the purpose of the readings, and if the explanation makes sense, there is nothing to complain about, unless, of course, you just want to whine, which is not very productive.

2. **Not taking time to clarify how student and supervisor evaluations will be done:** As far back as Chapter 2 we mentioned the importance of discussing grading criteria at the outset of the clinical practicum experience with your supervisor. You should be aware of exactly which clinical behaviors are important, your responsibilities, and how you will be graded. If possible, you should obtain a sample copy of an evaluation/grading form that will actually be used in the grading process. There is no excuse for arriving at the end of the semester and saying, "I didn't know that was important and I was being graded on it." Also, in almost every clinic, students are given the opportunity to evaluate the quality of clinical supervision that occurs during a semester. There is nothing wrong with discussing the behaviors that the supervisor will be "graded" on at the end of the term. If nothing else, it will bring to a conscious level in both the mind of the supervisor and the student what attributes are important in their practicum relationship.

3. **Failure to discuss the issue with the supervisor:** All the talking with students and other faculty members will not resolve a problem between your supervisor and you. It is always the best policy to go to your supervisor first to discuss any issue you are concerned about. This can be done in an organized and respectful manner, and in most cases the issue will be resolved in a positive way. Instead of wasting time talking to other people, go to your supervisor and say, "I was wondering if I might talk with you about a concern I have." We guarantee you that the

supervisor will be "all ears" and engage you in a discussion to resolve your problem. Now, it may not always be resolved the way you would prefer, but at least you have aired the issue and will receive a more detailed explanation of the supervisor's point of view. In the case of reading articles mentioned above, the supervisor might say, "The articles will show you how to do three specific tasks with your client, how to gather treatment data, and provide a good rationale for organizing your treatment plan, which is due next week." You still may not like reading the articles, but you've got to admit, the supervisor has some pretty good reasons to ask you to read them.

4. **Copying written materials from prior reports without thinking:** While in clinical practicum in the university clinic, you will often be assigned to work with a client who received treatment for several previous semesters. This client might also have been supervised by the same clinical faculty member during that time. Some students think that an easy thing to do is to simply copy the recommendations from the last report and turn those into a treatment plan. Sometimes these are copied verbatim from the previous semester's treatment report. There are several problems with this approach. First of all, the client may have changed since the last semester, especially if there has been a long break between terms. A second problem might be that you have a new supervisor taking over the case who may not agree with the recommendations. A third difficulty is that the information in prior reports might be wrong. We have seen, for example, students copy the same case history information section on a client over and over for a string of semesters. In one particular case, three successive reports written by different students stated that the client had normal hearing, when in fact it had never been screened due to lack of child cooperation in the evaluation. The supervisor never caught the error and signed the reports with the students who perpetuated the mistake. It is difficult to keep up with every detail of a client when you are supervising 20 different people. Also, once something is written down in a report, it tends to be treated as fact. Finally, and most important, if you merely copy a series of

recommendations or other report information, you have not really taken the opportunity to think about why goals were recommended or how assessment data were gathered. You have not gone through the process of problem solving but are just copying goals generated by someone else. Remember, part of the practicum experience is designed to help you learn to plan treatment in some principled way. Certainly, you should consider recommendations from the previous semester, but you should try to understand why they were made and come up with new considerations based on your knowledge from classroom work. In some cases, the supervisor may be ready to make some changes in the treatment program and your suggestions will be a breath of fresh air.

5. **Failure to take initiative:** Most students tend to do what they are told and not go "the extra mile." One way to really impress your supervisor is to come to a conference with some additional material that you have researched related to your client. This additional effort will be appreciated by most supervisors and show that you have a commitment to the case. Even if the supervisor does not want to incorporate the new material, it is something you might use with other clients, and it has shown that you have initiative.

6. **Failure to progressively assume more clinical responsibility:** As we illustrated in Figure 11-1, students should assume more clinical responsibility as they progress in practicum. Most supervisors will know where you are in terms of clinical development just by being aware of the cases you have worked with and the number of semesters of clinic you have completed. A major attribute the supervisor is looking for is your ability to apply your knowledge and previous experience to the current case. So if the student says, "I've worked with two other children at this level of language development. In those cases we developed a program like this (hands program to supervisor). I can modify this program with your input, or if you want to go a different direction, I would be happy to learn a new approach." Notice this shows that the student has ideas based on past experience and is willing to use them, modify them, or take a different direction. It shows

confidence, a reasoned approach to the case, and assumption of responsibility.

7. **Not being punctual for meetings and assignment deadlines:** A critical aspect of running *any type of clinical program in any setting* is making sure clinical sessions are started and completed on time and that paperwork deadlines are met. One of the most certain paths to a lower grade is to ignore deadlines and clinic schedules. There is no excuse for this, and if it happens to you it is important to acknowledge your error and try to never let it reoccur.

8. **Saying you understand when you don't:** Occasionally in a conference you will be told by your supervisor to incorporate a new task into treatment, but you do not understand what it is, how to do it, or why it is important. Some students in this situation will just nod their head, scribble down some notes, and never ask for clarification. They hope that talking to other students will clarify the issue or looking through class notes will assist them in understanding. It is almost always a losing strategy to not admit it when you are clueless. It is completely appropriate to say, "I was with you until you mentioned incorporating distinctive features into the therapy. Can you explain that a bit more, or tell me exactly where I might read about it before next week?" At least in this case you will get a more detailed explanation or a reference that will help you to design your therapy.

9. **Becoming frustrated with lack of client progress:** Everyone knows when a client is not making progress: the client, the family, the clinician, and the supervisor. Sometimes, the lack of progress goes along with a very severe disorder. Other times, it is possible that the treatment approach must be adjusted to result in more progress. If you are seeing your client over and over again, and the treatment data are not show-

ing any progress, then it is absolutely appropriate to ask your supervisor about this issue. You can say, "I've been working with John for 6 weeks now and he has not made any progress. Is this a typical pattern of response to therapy, or should we be thinking about changing our approach?" Chances are that the supervisor is just as frustrated as the student if the client is not making progress. If it is the case that this profile of client response is expected, the supervisor will tell you. If not, it is a good opportunity to rethink the approach and the supervisor will appreciate the chance to make adjustments. In this case, the student will be credited with being thoughtful and having initiative.

10. **Taking too much initiative when you are uncertain how to handle the situation:** Every student should be aware of his clinical limitations. If you have never done a procedure such as parent counseling, it would be inappropriate for you to engage in this without your supervisor's knowledge and consent. A good way to get into trouble is to come to a supervisory conference and say, "Oh, I counseled the parents on what to do at home for Charlie's stuttering." The supervisor might just indicate that such an occurrence is rather strange because the issue of a home program had never been discussed in conferences, and you have no experience with parent counseling. Always check with your supervisor before you engage in any procedure.

There are no doubt other communication issues and mistakes students can make with practicum supervisors. We have tried to give examples of common ones so the student can be proactive in interactions with clinical supervisors. As you can see, professional verbal communication is the medium by which problems with supervisors are confronted and solved. Keep those lines of communication open.

Appendices

Generator of Common Terms Used in Professional Communication*

The Person Receiving Services: Client, patient, child, student, the child's first name, use of a pronoun (he, she), Mr., Ms., or Mrs. followed by surname, the family, caretaker, spouse (wife/husband).

The Person Providing Services: The (this) clinician, speech-language pathologist, examiner, interventionist, evaluator, assessor, therapist.

Clinical Activity Completed: Treatment, remediation, intervention, rehabilitation, assessment, examination, testing, appraisal, diagnostic evaluation, counseling, training, therapy.

Parameters of Communication Involved:
Speech, communication, articulation, phonology, language, voice, fluency, hearing, swallowing.

Indicator of Disorder: Disorder, errors, abnormality, anomaly, deviation, difficulty, dysfunction, impairment, problem, disability, handicapping condition, deficit.

General "Professional Tone" Words

Ability, abilities	Adjustment
Administer, administered	Affect (emotion)
Appear, appears, appeared	Audiometric
Auditory acuity	Augmentative communication
Awareness	Baseline
Behavior	Bilingual
Caretaker	Case history

Causal	Characteristics, characterized
Clinical	Competency
Conduct, conducted	Congenital
Consistent, consistency	Demonstrate
Demonstrates, (ed)	Effect
Elderly	Eligibility, eligible
Environment	Etiology, etiological
Evidence, evidences, evidenced	Exhibited
Exhibits	Feedback
Feeding	Follow-up
Functional	Generalize, generalizes generalized
Goal, goals	Historically
Hospitalization, hospitalized	Identify, identified, identification
Impact	Improve, improves, improved
Impression, impressions	Increase, increases, increased
Indicate, indicates, indicated	Informant, informants
Intelligibility	Interview
Intonation	Inventory
Judgment	Level of performance
Limited, limitations	Manifest, manifests, manifested
Minimal	Multiple
Nature	Neonatal
Nonstandardized	Normative, norm-referenced
Objective, objectives	Observation

*Adapted from "The Agony of Report Writing: A New Look at an Old Problem," by W. O. Haynes and D. E. Hartman, 1975, *Journal of the National Student Speech and Hearing Association, 3*, pp. 7-15.

Occur, occurs, occurred
Oral
Outlook
Parent
Perform, performs, performed
Persistent
Precipitating factor
Prenatal

Production
Profound
Progress
Project, projects, projected
Psychometric
Rate
Reinforcement
Report, reports, reported
Response
Sample, sampling, sampled
Significant
Skill, skills
State, states, stated
Symptom, symptoms
Target behavior, behaviors
Terminate, terminated
Unremarkable
Valid

Verbalize, verbalizes, verbalized
Vocalize, vocalizations, vocalized

Onset
Organic
Parameter
Pediatric
Performance

Post-operative
Predisposing factor
Produce, produces, produced
Profile
Prognosis, prognostic
Progressive
Prosody, prosodic

Range
Refer, referral, referred
Reliable
Respond, responds, responded
Reveal, reveals, revealed
Severity

Significantly
Standardized
Status
Symptomatology
Task, tasks

Toddler
Utterance, utterances
Variable, variability, varied
Verbalization, verbalizations

Selected General Terms in Child Language

Bound morphemes
Caretaker-child interaction
Comprehension
Figurative language
Grammatical
Linguistic structures
Multiword
Play

Caretaker
Cohesion

Expressive
Gestural
Lexicon
Morphology
Narrative
Pragmatic

Processing, processes, processed
Repairs
Syntactic
Turn-taking Vocabulary

Receptive

Reciprocity
Topic manipulation
Word retrieval

Selected General Terms in Adult Language

Activities of daily living
Auditory comprehension
Brain injury
Closed head trauma
Coma
Dementia
Flaccid
Hemiparesis
Motor, motoric
Neurogenic
Paralysis
Premorbid
TBI
Word finding

Anomia
Bedside assessment
Circumlocution
Cognition
CVA
Executive function
Head injury
Lesion
Neglect
Neuromuscular
Paresis
Status post
Word retrieval

Selected General Terms in Voice Disorders

Abuse, misuse
Aerodynamic
Breath, breathing
Emission
Glottal, glottal attack
Loudness
Optimal
Phonation
Phonatory
Respiratory
Velopharyngeal, velopharyngeal closure
Voice
Vocal hygiene

Acoustic
Aphonia
Dysphonia
Frequency
Habitual
Nasality
Perceptual
Pitch
Resonance
Tracheoesophageal
Vocal

Vocal quality

Selected General Terms in Phonology

Phonological process
Production
Phoneme
Distinctive features
Phonetic context
Articulation
Omission
Distortion
Coarticulation, coarticulatory

Stimulability, stimulable
Phonetic placement
Phonemic
Phonological awareness
Misarticulation
Movement
Substitution
Syllable shape

Selected General Terms in Fluency

Dysfluency, dysfluencies dysfluent	Repetition
Prolongation	Hesitation
Block	Covert
Overt	Exteriorized
Interiorized	Pause
Filled pause	Avoidance
Rate	Secondary behavior(s)
Timing device	Adaptation
Consistency	Struggle
Circumlocution	

Selected General Terms for Dysphagia

Consistency	Aspiration
Liquids	Saliva

Chewing
Deglutition
Bolus
Transport
Regurgitation
Videofluoroscopic
Cough
Thin
Ground
Solids
Thin/thick
Oral transit
Nectar
Penetration
VSA
NPO

Swallow
Airway
Duration
Feeding
Oral intake
Positioning
Gagging
Pureed
Chopped
Barium swallow
Pooling
Mechanical soft diet
Honey
Pudding
FEES
MBS

Sample of University Clinic Diagnostic Report for Child Client Speech and Language Evaluation

Identifying Information

Name: Cameron Smith

D.O.B.: 1-1-04

Parent's Name: John & Amanda Smith

Address: 123 Maple St.
Yourtown, USA

Referred by: Dr. Samuel Jones

D.O.E.: 3-25-08

Age: 4.3

Tel: (123) 456-7890

Case History/Background Information

Cameron ("Cam") is a 4-year-old male who was referred to this clinic by his pediatrician, Dr. Samuel Jones, due to "unclear speech." According to parent report, Cam was delivered via caesarian section at 32 weeks gestation. He weighed 4 pounds, 2 ounces at birth, which is considered low birth weight. He remained hospitalized in the neonatal intensive care unit (NICU) for 5 weeks. His developmental milestones have all been delayed, as his mother reports that Cam did not start talking "until he was around 2 years old." Reportedly, he did not begin using multiword utterances until he was over 3 years. She also added that he did not walk until 13 months of age. Cam has a history of chronic ear infections, and was recently treated with a round of antibiotics. His mother stated that Cam is a happy child who is very outgoing, and "loves to talk." She also stated that people who are unfamiliar with Cam "don't understand anything he says."

Biological Bases of Communication

Cam's hearing was recently tested by his ENT and reported to be within normal limits. As part of today's evaluation, his hearing was screened at 1000, 2000, 4,000 Hz at 20 dB; results were normal. Based on cursory exam, Cam exhibits symmetrical facial features and normal movement and range of motion of the lips and tongue. Structure and function appear adequate for speech production.

Language

Clinical observation through play and formal testing were utilized to assess Cam's language skills. Cam easily engaged and established rapport with the clinicians. He demonstrated age-appropriate play and social interaction skills. The Preschool Language Scale (PLS-4) was administered to formally assess Cam's receptive and expressive language abilities. The results are as follows:

Auditory Comprehension

Raw Score: 50

Standard Score: 101 (53rd percentile)

Age-Equivalent: 3.10

Expressive Communication

Raw Score: 49

Standard Score: 92 (30th percentile)

Age-Equivalent: 4.0

Total Language Score: 96 (39th percentile)
Age-Equivalent: 4.1

Primary Area of Concern

Articulation

Based on the initial statement of the problem by Cam's parents, the focus of today's evaluation was on assessment of his articulation proficiency. Clinical observation and formal testing were utilized to assess Cam's articulation skills. According to the Goldman-Fristoe Test of Articulation (GFTA-2), Cam exhibits a significant articulation disorder, characterized by substitutions and omissions of sounds in all word positions. Following is a summary of his scores:

Raw Score: 28

Standard Score: 88 (21st percentile)

Age-Equivalent: 3.1

In addition, the Khan-Lewis Phonological Assessment (KLPA) was utilized to determine the extent to which Cam's articulation is affected by the use of phonological processes, or simplifications of the adult production of sounds. Cam was noted to reduce all consonant clusters and exhibit the following phonological processes: Stopping (p/f, b/v), Prevocalic Voicing (b/p, d/t), Gliding (w/r), and Assimilation ("guck" for "duck"). Three out of the four processes (Stopping, Cluster Reduction, Gliding) commonly persist in children with speech deficits past the age of 3. It should be noted that Cam was not stimulable for any sounds produced in error during the evaluation. For this reason, speech therapy to address correct production of age-appropriate phonemes is warranted. His overall intelligibility in connected speech is judged to be approximately 50% to an untrained familiar listener.

Voice/Fluency

Voice and fluency are judged to be within normal limits at this time.

Pragmatics

Cam is a friendly little boy who enjoys social interaction. He initiates conversation and responds appropriately to questions during play as well as structured language activities.

Clinical Impressions and Recommendations

Cam is a 4-year-old male with a remarkable medical history, including premature birth and developmental delays. He presents today with a severe articulation disorder that significantly affects his ability to communicate. Receptive and expressive language, voice, and fluency are within normal limits at this time. It is felt that Cam would benefit from speech therapy to address the aforementioned articulation deficits. Goals should include the following:

1. Improved production of fricatives /f/ and /v/
2. Improved production of voiceless stops /p/, /t/ in prevocalic position
3. Reduction of assimilation process targeting age-appropriate phonemes

Sample of University Clinic Diagnostic Report for Adult Client Speech and Language Evaluation

Identifying Information

Name: Jane Adams   **Date of Evaluation:** 2-22-07

D.O.B.: 6-20-35   **Age:** 71

Address: 123 Oak St.   **Telephone:** (456) 123-5678
City, USA

Referred by: Spouse   **Physician:** Steve Powers, M.D.

Case History/Presenting Complaint

Jane Adams is a 69-year-old retired female who was referred to this clinic by her spouse, in order to improve her expressive language skills and short-term memory. Mrs. Adams suffered a left hemisphere cerebrovascular accident (CVA) approximately 3 months ago. Her husband reports that her symptoms began the afternoon of November 26, 2006, with Mrs. Adams' complaints of being "confused." The next morning, he awoke to find her using "slurred speech" and with right-sided weakness. She was admitted to the hospital and was later transferred to the Regional Rehabilitation Center, where she remained for 2 weeks. Her physician, Dr. Powers, reported that MRI revealed an acute infarct in the posterior cerebral artery territory, as well as old lacunar infarcts. She received intensive speech, occupational, and physical therapy during her 2 weeks at the rehabilitation hospital. Mrs. Adams has a history of osteoporosis, and is now taking the following medications: Fosamax, Aspirin, Vytorin, and a multivitamin. She is now ambulatory and uses a quad cane when walking longer distances.

Biological Bases of Communication

Vision/Hearing

Mrs. Adams reports no change to her vision or hearing since her stroke. Her vision is aided with eyeglasses.

Oral/Facial Examination

Mrs. Adams exhibits symmetrical facial features, and does not demonstrate or report any signs of facial weakness; however, her ability to produce rapid alternating movements is mildly impaired for repeated productions of /pu, tu, ku/. She reports that she is able to manage a regular diet at this time. Lingual and labial coordination and range of motion are grossly within normal limits. Overall, structure and function are adequate for speech production.

Primary Area of Concern

Language

The Western Aphasia Battery–Revised (WAB) was administered on February 2, 2007. The WAB is a diagnostic instrument used to evaluate the following clinical aspects of language function: content, fluency, auditory comprehension, repetition and naming, reading, writing, and calculation (Kertesz & Poole, 1974). The supplemental reading, writing, and calculation sections were not administered during this evaluation. According to the results of the assessment, Mrs. Adams exhibits a moderate anomic aphasia, or an inability to supply words for what she wants to talk about, specifically significant nouns and verbs. The results of testing are as follows.

Spontaneous Speech

Conversational Questions: 2/6

Picture Description: Some grammatical organization, marked word-finding difficulty

Auditory Verbal Comprehension

Yes/No Questions: 54/60

Auditory Word Recognition: 58/60

Sequential Commands: 70/80

Repetition

Words and Sentences: 96/100

Naming and Word Finding

Object Naming: 24/60

Word Fluency: 2/20

Sentence Completion: 8/10

Responsive Speech: 7/10

Aphasia Quotient: 65.6/100 (Moderate)

Although she does not exhibit any signs of apraxia or dysarthria, Mrs. Adams does exhibit difficulty expressing herself in complete sentences due to her aphasia. According to the speech pathologist who treated her in the rehab hospital, Mrs. Adams "continues to display anomia and moderate to severe expressive deficits that are most evident at the conversational level."

Articulation

There were no articulation errors noted during the evaluation. Mrs. Adams' speech is judged to be 100% intelligible to a familiar or unfamiliar listener.

Voice/Fluency

Mrs. Adams exhibits age- and gender-appropriate vocal quality; speech is somewhat dysfluent due to her frequent hesitations, restarts, and word finding difficulties. She does not exhibit, nor does she report, any stuttering presently or prior to her stroke.

Pragmatics

Mrs. Adams has fair conversational skills. She is able to initiate, take appropriate turns, and briefly maintain a topic; however, she has difficulty participating in a conversation due to her expressive aphasia. During conversation she frequently remarked, "Oh my gosh, now I just had it."

continues

Clinical Impressions and Recommendations

Jane Adams is a 69–year-old female who suffered a left hemisphere CVA in November 2006. She presents today with mild to moderate anomic aphasia. Voice, fluency, and articulation are within normal limits at this time. It is recommended that Mrs. Adams receive speech therapy twice per week for 1-hour sessions. Goals for treatment should continue to focus on expressive language and memory tasks such as:

1. Picture description using sentences
2. Naming 3 steps in completing an everyday task
3. Listening to a short story and answering "wh" questions
4. Recalling details from a short narrative
5. Role play with clinician of everyday activities, such as ordering in a restaurant, following a recipe, doing laundry
6. Demonstrate knowledge of compensatory strategies for anomia and short-term memory deficits.

Example of a Communication Addendum from a Medical Facility

Total Visits from SOC _____ Total cancellations/no show _____

HEALTHSOUTH ®

Facility Name: _____

UPDATED PLAN OF CARE (≥ 60 days) SPEECH-LANGUAGE PATHOLOGY

ADDRESSOGRAPH

Patient Name: _____ Onset Date: _____ Begin Date: _____

Primary Diagnosis: _____ Prior hospitalization (for current episode): From _____ to _____ ☐ N/A

Treatment Diagnosis(es): _____

Physician: _____

Rehab potential: ☐ Excellent ☐ Good ☐ Fair   Certification period: From _____ To _____

☐ Completed Medication/Diagnosis Update Form

Summary of Progress (Progress achieved from previously stated goals)

_____
_____
_____
_____

Short term goals are written to address patient problems and should relate to long term goals.

Short Term Goals: _____ Weeks

1. Patient will: _____
2. Patient will: _____
3. Patient will: _____
4. Patient will: _____
5. Patient will: _____

Long Term Goals: _____ Weeks

1. ☐ Express basic needs/wants via single words/phrases/gestures/ augmentative communication
2. ☐ Converse in small group settings with familiar listeners
3. ☐ Yes/No reliability to facilitate care
4. ☐ Follow simple directions (with or without cues) for ADL's
5. ☐ Comprehension adequate for ADL's with caregiver
6. ☐ Able to follow logical sequences to complete ADL's
7. ☐ Able to identify and solve basic problems related to ADL's/ vocational needs
8. ☐ Speech intelligible to caregivers at word/phrase level
9. ☐ Perform oral-motor exercise program independently to maximize strength and ROM of oral musculature for speech/swallowing.
10. ☐ Reading comprehension for safety (ie. labels, directions) with ADL's in home
11. ☐ Independently utilize speech intelligibility strategies to maximize skills of verbal expression in community/environment.

12. ☐ Reading comprehension for paragraph length material
13. ☐ Calculation for time management with household ADL's
14. ☐ Gross accuracy of numerical processing with basic problems of everyday living
15. ☐ Normalization of swallow with or without compensatory techniques with safe oral intake to consume _____% of meals.
16. ☐ Patient able to use compensatory strategies for basic ADL's
17. ☐ Writing legible for ADL's ie. notes/checks
18. ☐ Attention to functional tasks in daily environment
19. ☐ Recall daily events via compensatory strategies
20. ☐ Other _____
21. ☐ Other _____
22. ☐ Other _____
23. ☐ Other _____
24. ☐ Other _____

Patient Goals: _____
_____

Treatment Plan: Skilled intervention may include the following:

☐ Communication   ☐ Voice   ☐ Home Exercise Program
☐ Swallowing   ☐ Aural rehab   ☐ Patient/Family training
☐ Cognitive retraining   ☐ Work re-entry ☐ Other _____
☐ Patient/caregiver participation   ☐ School re-entry
   in development of treatment plan.

Treatment Frequency: _____ Times/Week **Duration:** _____ Weeks

I have received this Plan of Care and have seen this patient and re-certify a continuing need for services.

Physician Signature _____ **Date** _____

Therapist Signature _____ **Date** _____

My therapist has reviewed my Plan of Care with me. **Patient/Caregiver Signature** _____

Revised 3/04   Page 1 of 1   ©HRC 2003
(Form meets HCFA 701 requirements)   394 - UPDATED PLAN OF CARE SPEECH-LANGUAGE PATHOLOGY

Appendix D. Communication Addendum from a Rehabilitation Hospital. (Used with Permission from Healthsouth Corporation.)

Example of a Cognitive Addendum from a Medical Facility

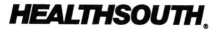

INTERDISCIPLINARY ASSESSMENT

COGNITIVE ADDENDUM	
Severity Rating: Use these ratings on the lines below. Independent- 100% Accuracy (IND) Modified Indep. -WFL/ 100% with assistive device or extra time (MOD I) Supervision -requires assistance less than 10% (SPV) Minimally impaired 75 - 90% accuracy (MIN) Moderately impaired 50 - 74% accuracy (MOD) Severely impaired 25 - 49 % accuracy (SEV) Profoundly impaired 0 - 24% accuracy (PRO) NT= Not tested	**Cognitive Diagnosis:** **Anticipated Functional Outcomes:** **Rancho Level: (If Applicable)**
LEVEL OF ALERTNESS: (Check One) ____ Alert / Focused ____ Alert / Unfocused / Inattentive ____ Lethargic / Somnolent ____ Unresponsive ____ Inconsistent	**PROBLEM SOLVING / REASONING:** Overall Severity Rating_ _____ Simple nonverbal reasoning ____ Complex nonverbal reasoning ____ Simple verbal reasoning ____ Abstract / complex verbal reasoning ____ Mathematical skills:_____
ATTENTION: Overall Severity Rating_____ ____ Sustained attention to task in 1:1 environment (> 3 minutes) ____ Selective attention in distracting environment ____ Alternating attention between more than one task ____ Divided attention in distracting environment	**ORIENTATION:** Overall Severity Rating_ ____ ____ Person (Name) ____ Place (Building, City, State) ____ Time (Year, Month, Day, Date) ____ Situation
MEMORY: Overall Severity Rating_____ ____ Recalls biographical information Verbal Visual Immediate Memory _____ _____ Short Term Memory _____ _____ Long Term Memory _____ _____ Procedural Memory _____ _____	**EXECUTIVE FUNCTION:** Overall Severity Rating_ ____ ____ Initiation ____ Goal Setting ____ Organization ____ Planning / Decision Making ____ Self Monitoring ____ Time Management

INSIGHT: (Check All That Apply)
❏ Demonstrates awareness of current limitations / deficits
❏ Expresses need for assistance
❏ Demonstrates ability to compensate for deficits
	SAFETY AWARENESS: (Check All That Apply)
	❏ Demonstrates awareness of needs for safety precautions
	    during functional situation.
	❏ Demonstrates use of safety precautions during functional
	    situation.
	❏ Unaware of safety precautions during functional situations.

REFERRAL / TREATMENT: (Check All That Apply) ❏ Behavioral Program ❏ Formal Neuropsych Evaluation ❏ Referral for treatment of above deficits ❏ Other	**BEHAVIORAL / MOTIVATION:** (Check All That Apply) ❏ Impulsive ❏ Agitated / Aggressive ❏ Perseveration ❏ Other
SPECIAL TESTING:	
COMMENTS:	
Signature / Title	Date:

Appendix E. Cognitive Addendum from a Rehabilitation Hospital. (Used with permission from Healthsouth Corporation.)

Example of a Dysphagia Addendum from a Medical Facility

HEALTHSOUTH ®

Facility Name: _____

DYSPHAGIA ADDENDUM

☐ Initial   ☐ Re-eval   ☐ D/C _____

CURRENT DIET: _____

SWALLOWING HISTORY: _____
_____
_____
_____
_____
_____
_____

PREVIOUS MBS: ☐ YES   ☐ NO   DATE/RESULTS: _____

GENERAL OBSERVATIONS:

A. Patient Positioning: ☐ Upright In Chair   ☐ Other _____
B. Alertness: ☐ Alert   ☐ Lethargic   ☐ Inconsistent
C. Behavior: ☐ Distractible   ☐ Noncompliant   ☐ Impulsive
D. Commun./Cognitive Status: ☐ Memory WFL   ☐ Follows Simple Commands
    ☐ Verbalizes Needs   ☐ Receptive Language Deficits
    ☐ Expressive Aphasia   ☐ Apraxia
E. Oral Motor
    Labial   ☐ Adequate   ☐ Inadequate _____
    Lingual   ☐ Adequate   ☐ Inadequate _____
    Cough/Throat Clear   ☐ Adequate   ☐ Inadequate _____
    Dry Swallow   ☐ Adequate   ☐ Inadequate _____
    Facial Symmetry   ☐ L / R Facial Droop   ☐ Hypertonicity
F. Dentition   ☐ Full Dentures   ☐ Partial Dentures   ☐ Missing Teeth   ☐ Malocclusion
G. Trach: ☐ No   ☐ Yes   Type/Size _____
    (During Exam)   ☐ Inflated   ☐ Deflated   ☐ Capped   ☐ Uncapped

Check, if apply:	Difficulty Chewing L / R / B	Pocketing L / R / B	Increased Oral Transit Time	Bolus Formation Difficulty	Coughing	Change In Vocal Quality	Delayed Swallowing	Decreased Laryngeal Evaluation	Other
Puree									
Ground									
Mechanical Soft									
Chopped									
Regular									
Thin Liquid									
Nectar Thick									
Honey Thick									

RECOMMENDATIONS:

Diet Consistency: Solids: _____ Liquids: _____ NPO: _____
Medications: ☐ Non Oral ☐ Crushed ☐ Liquid ☐ Whole _____
Level of Supervision: ☐ 1 - 1 by _____ ☐ Feeding Group   ☐ Intermittent   ☐ None

STRATEGIES - FOODS:
☐ Place Food in R / L Side   ☐ Multiple Swallow
☐ Chin Down   ☐ Quiet Environment
☐ Encourage Chewing   ☐ Turn/Tilt Head L / R
☐ Small bites   ☐ Slow Rate
☐ Check For Pocketing   ☐ Tilt Head Back
☐ Discourage Talking   ☐ Alternate Food/Liquid
   While Eating   ☐ Other:

STRATEGIES - LIQUID:
☐ Spoon Only   ☐ Multiple Swallow
☐ From Cup   ☐ No Straw
☐ Small Sips   ☐ Use Straw
☐ Chin Down   ☐ Turn / Tilt Head L / R
☐ Other _____

ADDITIONAL ASSESSMENT/CONSULTATIONS:
☐ Instrumental Assessment _____
☐ Follow-up Clinical Assessment on _____
☐ Dysphagia Therapy

☐ Dietician Consultation   ☐ Oral Motor Regime
☐ Self Feeding Referral   ☐ Speech / Language
☐ Other _____   Evaluation & Treat

Date	Signature / Title	Date	Signature / Title

Appendix F. Cognitive Addendum from a Rehabilitation Hospital. (Used with permission from Healthsouth Corporation.)

Example of an Eligibility Form Used in Public Schools

NOTICE AND ELIGIBILITY DECISION
REGARDING SPECIAL EDUCATION SERVICES

STUDENT'S NAME: _____

Date Notice of Eligibility Decision Given or Sent to Parent/Student (Age 19): 06/24/2005 _____

Check One:	☐ Initial Eligibility ☐ Reevaluation		
AREA OF ASSESSMENT	**DATE OF ASSESSMENT**	**NAME OF ASSESSMENT AND RESULTS**	**STRENGTHS/NEEDS OF CHILD**

Appendix G. Eligibility Form from the Public School Setting. (Used with permission from Alabama State Department of Education.) *(continues)*

Student's Name

AREA OF ASSESSMENT	DATE OF ASSESSMENT	NAME OF ASSESSMENT AND RESULTS	STRENGTHS/NEEDS OF CHILD

Appendix G. *(continues)*

Student's Name

<table>
<tr><td rowspan="2">FOR
LD
ONLY</td><td>1. Severe discrepancy (SD) between ability and achievement:</td><td>☐ YES   ☐ NO</td></tr>
</table>

1. Severe discrepancy (SD) between ability and achievement: ☐ YES   ☐ NO

    A. If using the predicted achievement (regression to the mean) model (effective 7/1/98):

      • IQ score: _____

      • Predicted Achievement (PA) Score: _____

      • Obtained Achievement (OA) score(s):

PA <u>00</u> - OA <u>00</u> = SD <u>00</u>	
PA <u>00</u> - OA <u>00</u> = SD <u>00</u>	
(SD must be 16 or greater for all ages)	

         One Total Score: _____

          or

     Two Subtest/Two Composite
     Scores from two different tests: _____   _____

    B. If using simple standard score method (for students identified before July 1, 1998):

IQ Score _____ - Achievement Score _____ = SD 00 _____   (SD must be 15 or greater to 11 years; must be 23 or greater for 11 years and older)

2. For educationally relevant behaviors noted during the classroom observation(s) and educationally relevant medical findings (if any), please refer to page _____ of this report.

3. Relationship of the educationally relevant behaviors to the student's academic functioning is:
_____

4. The following factors have been ruled out as the primary cause of the impairment (check all that apply):
    ☐ Environmental/Cultural/Economic Concerns   ☐ Visual/Hearing Disabilities
    ☐ Mental Retardation   ☐ Emotional Disturbance   ☐ Motor Disabilities

Was the student's lack of instruction in math or reading or the student's limited English proficiency a determining factor in the decision?   ☐ **YES**   ☐ **NO**

ELIGIBILITY DECISION

ELIGIBLE: ☐ YES   ☐ NO   AREA OF DISABILITY: _____

Explanation (if needed)

DESCRIPTION OF OTHER OPTIONS CONSIDERED AND WHY THEY WERE REJECTED, IF APPLICABLE

Appendix G. *(continues)*

Student's Name

ELIGIBILITY TEAM MEMBERS			

	NAME	POSITION	DATE
I **AGREE** with the conclusions written in this report.	_____	_____	_____
	_____	_____	_____
	_____	_____	_____
	_____	_____	_____
	_____	_____	_____
	_____	_____	_____
	_____	_____	_____
	_____	_____	_____

	NAME	POSITION	DATE
I **DO NOT AGREE** with the conclusions written in this report. The attached statement represents my conclusions in this area.	_____	_____	_____
	_____	_____	_____
	_____	_____	_____
	_____	_____	_____
	_____	_____	_____
	_____	_____	_____
	_____	_____	_____
	_____	_____	_____
	_____	_____	_____

My signature below verifies that if you require notice and an explanation of your rights in your native language, you have been accommodated to ensure your understanding. You are fully protected under the rights addressed in your copy of the *Special Education Rights* document. If you would like another copy of these rights, have any questions, or wish to schedule a conference, please contact:

Name: _____   Telephone: _____

Sincerely,

_____
Signature of Education Agency Official

Appendix G. *(continued)*

Example of University Clinic Daily Treatment Plan

DAILY THERAPY PLAN

Client: K.W. **File Number:** 00-123-98
Clinician: R. Smith **Supervisor:** Haynes
Disorder: Language **Date:** 7-13-07

STO 1: The client will imitate productions of short phrases and sentences during structured play activities with 80% accuracy.

Procedure: The clinician and client will engage in a variety of structured play activities using high interest toys such as farm animals, Mr. Potato Head, and books. The clinician will model phrases and sentences during play such as, "cow in barn," or "I want more," and instruct the client to imitate.

STO 2: The client will correctly respond to "wh" questions using "what" and "where" with 90% accuracy during structured play activities.

Procedure: The clinician will ask the client "what" and "where" questions during joint book reading and play with toys.

STO 3: The client will increase requesting for desired objects to at least 10 times with minimal prompting during a 45-minute session.

Procedure: The clinician will prompt the client to request desired objects when playing with cars, Mr. Potato Head, and play-doh.

Example of a Plan of Care from a Medical Facility

Total Visits from SOC _____ Total cancellations/no show _____

HEALTHSOUTH®

Facility Name: _____

UPDATED PLAN OF CARE (≥ 60 days) SPEECH-LANGUAGE PATHOLOGY

Patient Name: _____ Onset Date: _____ ~~ADDRESSOGRAPH~~ Begin Date: _____

Primary Diagnosis: _____ Prior hospitalization (for current episode): From _____ to _____ ☐ N/A

Treatment Diagnosis(es): _____

Physician: _____

Rehab potential: ☐ Excellent ☐ Good ☐ Fair   Certification period: From _____ To _____

☐ Completed Medication/Diagnosis Update Form

Summary of Progress (Progress achieved from previously stated goals)

_____
_____
_____
_____

Short term goals are written to address patient problems and should relate to long term goals.

Short Term Goals: _____ Weeks

1. Patient will: _____
2. Patient will: _____
3. Patient will: _____
4. Patient will: _____
5. Patient will: _____

Long Term Goals: _____ Weeks

1. ☐ Express basic needs/wants via single words/phrases/gestures/ augmentative communication
2. ☐ Converse in small group settings with familiar listeners
3. ☐ Yes/No reliability to facilitate care
4. ☐ Follow simple directions (with or without cues) for ADL's
5. ☐ Comprehension adequate for ADL's with caregiver
6. ☐ Able to follow logical sequences to complete ADL's
7. ☐ Able to identify and solve basic problems related to ADL's/ vocational needs
8. ☐ Speech intelligible to caregivers at word/phrase level
9. ☐ Perform oral-motor exercise program independently to maximize strength and ROM of oral musculature for speech/swallowing.
10. ☐ Reading comprehension for safety (ie. labels, directions) with ADL's in home
11. ☐ Independently utilize speech intelligibility strategies to maximize skills of verbal expression in community/environment.

12. ☐ Reading comprehension for paragraph length material
13. ☐ Calculation for time management with household ADL's
14. ☐ Gross accuracy of numerical processing with basic problems of everyday living
15. ☐ Normalization of swallow with or without compensatory techniques with safe oral intake to consume _____% of meals.
16. ☐ Patient able to use compensatory strategies for basic ADL's
17. ☐ Writing legible for ADL's ie. notes/checks
18. ☐ Attention to functional tasks in daily environment
19. ☐ Recall daily events via compensatory strategies
20. ☐ Other _____
21. ☐ Other _____
22. ☐ Other _____
23. ☐ Other _____
24. ☐ Other _____

Patient Goals: _____
_____

Treatment Plan: Skilled intervention may include the following:

☐ Communication
☐ Swallowing
☐ Cognitive retraining
☐ Patient/caregiver participation in development of treatment plan.

☐ Voice
☐ Aural rehab
☐ Work re-entry
☐ School re-entry

☐ Home Exercise Program
☐ Patient/Family training
☐ Other _____

Treatment Frequency: _____ Times/Week   **Duration:** _____ Weeks

I have received this Plan of Care and have seen this patient and re-certify a continuing need for services.

Physician Signature _____   **Date** _____

Therapist Signature _____   **Date** _____

My therapist has reviewed my Plan of Care with me.   **Patient/Caregiver Signature** _____

Revised 3/04   Page 1 of 1   ©HRC 2003
(Form meets HCFA 701 requirements)   394 - UPDATED PLAN OF CARE SPEECH-LANGUAGE PATHOLOGY

Appendix I. Plan of Care from a Rehabilitation Hospital Setting. (Used with permission from Healthsouth Corporation.)

List of Selected Medical Abbreviations Used in Paperwork

ADLs—activities of daily living

Ax—assessment

A—assistance

Δ—change

C/O —complains of

↓—decreased

Dx—diagnosis

Hx—history

↑—increased

L—left

Max—maximum

Min—minimum

Mod—moderate

Mod-A—moderate assistance

NG—nasogastric (feeding tube placed in the nose)

NPO—"nothing per oral," or no oral feeding

OMEs—oral motor exercises

P—prompts

PEG—percutaneous endoscopic gastrostomy (feeding tube placed in the stomach)

POC—plan of care

PRN—per necessary, or when needed

Pt—Patient

R—right

R/O—rule out

ROM—range of motion

2—secondary to

Tx—therapy

p̱—with

s̄—without

Example of an IFSP Used in Preschool Settings

INDIVIDUALIZED FAMILY SERVICE PLAN

Connecticut
Birth to Three
System

*Date: _____

*Type of meeting: ☐ Interim IFSP ☐ Initial IFSP ☐ Annual ☐ Review

*Child's Name: _____

*Date of Birth: _____

☐ *Male
☐ *Female

Parent/Foster Parent/Guardian/Family Member (circle one)	Parent/Guardian/Family Member (circle one)
*Name	*Name
*Address	*Address
*City *State *Zip	*City *State *Zip
*Phone (day) (Evening)	*Phone (day) (Evening)
*Primary Language	*Primary Language

*Surrogate Parent: _____   *Phone: _____

*Address: _____

*Service Coordinator/Program: _____   *Phone: _____

*Address: _____

*Physician/Health Care Provider: _____   *Phone: _____

*Address: _____

*School District: _____ Contact Person/Phone: _____

*Recommended school district referral date, no later than: _____ date
(Refer the child any time after the 2nd birthday. The decision to refer must be made no later than age 2 1/2)

*Denotes part of the electronic record _____ date

☐ *Check if release to LEA (form 3-3) is on file
☐ *Check if referral to LEA (form 3-8) is on file

Connecticut Birth to Three Form 3-1 (Revised 7/1/06)   Confidential Document

Appendix K. Example of an Individualized Family Service Plan (IFSP). (Used with Permission from Connecticut Birth to Three System.) *(continues)*

Child's Name: _____ DOB: _____ Date: _____

SECTION I. SUMMARY OF CHILD'S PRESENT ABILITIES, STRENGTHS, AND NEEDS

1. Indicate the dates and types of evaluation or assessment report, which were used to develop this plan:

_____

_____

2. Summarize below additional observations by family and other team members of the child's abilities, strengths, and needs in daily routines. Areas to include:

- What are your child's likes and dislikes?
- What are your child's frustrations?
- How does your child spend his/her day?

- Bathing, feeding, dressing, toileting – Adaptive/Self help skills
- Thinking, reasoning and learning – Cognitive skills
- Moving, hearing, vision, health – Physical development
- Feelings, coping, getting along with others – Social/Emotional development
- Understanding, communicating with others and expressing self with others – Communication skills

_____

_____

_____

_____

_____

_____

_____

_____

_____

_____

_____

_____

(Attach additional pages as needed)

Connecticut Birth to Three Form 3-1 (Revised 7/1/06)

Appendix K. (*continues*)

Child's Name: _____ DOB: _____ Date: _____

SECTION II. SUMMARY OF FAMILY'S CONCERNS, PRIORITIES, AND RESOURCES
AS THEY RELATE TO ENHANCING THEIR CHILD'S DEVELOPMENT - Family Outcome

1. Information about our family for the IFSP: (Suggestions)

- Things we like to do as a family
- Who is part of our family?
- Important events that have occurred
- People and agencies we find helpful.
- Our family's strengths in meeting our child's needs.
- How our child's special needs affect our family

2. What would be helpful for our family in the months and year ahead? (Family Outcome)

3. What assistance or information will we need to achieve this outcome? (Strategies)

SECTION III. OTHER SERVICES THAT ARE IN PLACE OR ARE NEEDED

Services such as medical, recreational, religious, social and other child related services, not covered by the CT Birth to Three System, that contribute to this plan.

Resource/Program/Support Service	✓ If Needed	Payment Source

Connecticut Birth to Three Form 3-1 (Revised 7/1/06)

Confidential Document

Appendix K. *(continues)*

Child's Name: _____ DOB: _____ Date: _____

SECTION IV. PLAN FOR TRANSITION FROM THE BIRTH TO THREE SYSTEM
TO PRESCHOOL SPECIAL EDUCATION OR OTHER APPROPRIATE SERVICES

1. Information that would be helpful for our child and family to plan for the future. • Community program options • LEA information • Referral process • Rights and responsibilities
• Parent training • Visiting community programs • Adaptive equipment • Transportation • Time with other children • Information sharing.

2. What are the next steps?	Who will be involved:	Date to be completed:

After the initial IFSP meeting, this plan may only be modified at an IFSP periodic review meeting or annual IFSP meeting

Connecticut Birth to Three Form 3-1 (Revised 7/1/06)

Appendix K. *(continues)*

Child's Name: _____ DOB: _____ Date: _____

SECTION V. OUTCOME #___

What we want is: _____

What is happening now: _____

_____

What are the next steps (objectives) to reach this outcome?

	Expected timeframe for reaching objective

Strategies: methods for working on this outcome during your child and family's daily activities and routines

	People who will be involved

(Attach additional pages as needed)

Connecticut Birth to Three Form 3-1 (Revised 7/1/06)

Appendix K. *(continues)*

Child's Name: _____ DOB: _____ Date: _____

SECTION VI. EARLY INTERVENTION SERVICES AND SUPPORTS

*What is going to happen (including assistive technology)	*Delivered by: (Discipline responsible)	*Location	*How Often	*How Long	*Start Date	*End Date
		Code				

☐ Check here if additional pages are attached to list or clarify the services being provided or the schedule of services.

Primary service location codes: 1=home 2=setting designed for typical children 3=hospital (inpatient) 4=residential facility 5=service provider office 6=setting designed for children with delays 7=other

☐ *Check if any early intervention service cannot be achieved satisfactorily in a natural environment and attach a justification for each service.

Informed Consent by Parents. Check and sign below:

1. _____ I understand my rights under this program and received a written copy of *Parent Rights Under IDEA Part C* **and**

   or

2a. _____ I give permission to carry out this Individualized Family Service Plan as written.

2b. _____ I do not accept this Individualized Family Service Plan as written, however I do give permission for the following services to begin:

Services are paid for by the **Birth to Three System** unless otherwise indicated:
Service Coordinator/ Discipline/ Program Name/phone #:
Service Coordination is provided to all families at least monthly and is most often part of the early intervention visit

Parent Signature _____ Date _____ Parent Signature _____

I have reviewed this Individualized Family Service Plan, which is based in part on an evaluation in all areas of development. I confirm the appropriateness of the diagnosis(es) as stated by the diagnostic (ICD-9) code and the recommendations for the treatment services as they are written.

Physician Signature: _____ LIC#: _____ *Date: _____

*Print Name: _____ *ICD-9 Code(s) _____

*Denotes part of the electronic record

Connecticut Birth to Three Form 3-1 (Revised 7/1/06)

Parent Signature _____ Date _____

Appendix K. *(continues)*

Confidential Document

Child's Name: _____ DOB: _____ Date: _____

SECTION VII. IFSP TEAM MEMBERS

The following individuals have participated in the development of the IFSP and/or will assist in its implementation. There will be ongoing verbal communication between the IFSP team members listed below to assist in the implementation of the IFSP.

Name	Relationship	Phone	Method of participation

Meeting Notes: (discussion, specific scheduling issues, and any other issues)

Connecticut Birth to Three Form 3-1 (Revised 7/1/06)

Appendix K. *(continues)*

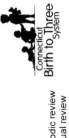

Connecticut
Birth to Three System

Section R-1: Individualized Family Service Plan (IFSP) Review: Outcomes

Child's Name: _____ DOB: _____ Review Date: _____ ☐ Periodic review ☐ Annual review

Date of IFSP being reviewed: _____ Reason for review: _____

Outcome #	Outcome(s)	Progress towards reaching *family* outcomes	Status

Outcome #	Outcome(s)	Progress towards reaching *child* outcomes	Status

Progress on Transition Plan

Attach additional pages as needed and additional outcomes if developed.

Connecticut Birth to Three Form 3-1 (Revised 7/1/06)

Confidential Document

Appendix K. *(continues)*

171

Section R-2 Individualized Family Service Plan (IFSP) Review: Services and Supports

Child's Name: _____ DOB: _____ Date of IFSP being reviewed: _____ Review Date: _____

Result of Review: _____

SUMMARY OF REVISED EARLY INTERVENTION SERVICES AND SUPPORTS
(To be completed after review of outcomes)

*What is going to happen (including assistive technology)	*Delivered by: (Discipline responsible)	*Location code	*How Often	*How Long	*Start Date	*End Date

☐ Check here if additional pages are attached to list or clarify the services being provided or the schedule of services.

Primary service location codes: 1=home 2=setting designed for typical children 3=hospital (inpatient) 4=residential facility 5=service provider office 6=setting designed for children with delays 7=other

☐ *Check if any early intervention service cannot be achieved satisfactorily in a natural environment and attach a justification for each service.

Services are paid for by the Birth to Three System unless otherwise indicated:

Service Coordinator/Program/Discipline/phone#:
_____

Service Coordination is provided to all families at least monthly and is most often part of the early intervention visit

Informed Consent by Parents. Check and sign below:

1. _____ I understand my rights under this program and received a written copy of *Parent Rights Under IDEA Part C* **and**

2a. _____ I give permission to carry out this Individualized Family Service Plan as written.

or

2b. _____ I do not accept this Individualized Family Service Plan as written, however I do give permission for the following services to begin:

Parent Signature _____ Date _____ Parent Signature _____

I have reviewed the revisions made to this Individualized Family Service Plan. I confirm the appropriateness of the diagnosis(es) as stated by the diagnostic (ICD-9) code and the recommendations for the treatment services as they are written.

Physician Signature: _____ LIC#: _____ *Date: _____

*Print Name: _____ *ICD-9 Code(s) _____ , _____ , _____

*Denotes part of the electronic record

Connecticut Birth to Three Form 3-1 (Revised 7/1/06)

Appendix K. *(continues)*

Child's Name: _____ DOB: _____ Date: _____

JUSTIFICATION FOR EARLY INTERVENTION SERVICES THAT CANNOT BE ACHIEVED SATISFACTORILY IN A NATURAL ENVIRONMENT

LOCATION OF SERVICE: _____ SERVICE: _____

1. Explain how and why the child's outcome(s) could not be met if the service were provided in the child's natural environment with supplementary supports. If the child has not made satisfactory progress towards an outcome in a natural environment, include a description of why alternative natural environments have not been selected or outcome not modified.	
2. Explain how services provided in this location will be generalized to support the child's ability to function in his or her natural environment.	
3. Describe a plan with timelines and supports necessary to allow the child's outcome(s) to be satisfactorily achieved in his or her natural environment.	

Child's Name: _____ DOB: _____ Date: _____

ADDITIONAL PAGE
INDIVIDUALIZED FAMILY SERVICE PLAN

_____

_____

_____

_____

_____

_____

_____

_____

_____

_____

_____

_____

_____

_____

_____

_____

_____

_____

_____

_____

Connecticut Birth to Three Form 3-1 (Revised 1/1/06)

Appendix K. *(continues)*

Example of an IEP Used in Public School Settings

INDIVIDUALIZED EDUCATION PROGRAM

STUDENT'S NAME: _____

DOB _____ SCHOOL YEAR _____ - _____ GRADE _____ - _____

IEP INITIATION/DURATION DATES   FROM _____ TO _____

THIS IEP WILL BE IMPLEMENTED DURING THE REGULAR SCHOOL TERM UNLESS NOTED IN EXTENDED SCHOOL YEAR SERVICES.

STUDENT PROFILE

Page _____ of _____

SDE Approved 5/22/2007

Appendix L. Example of an Individual Educational Program (IEP) Used in Public School Settings. (Used with permission from the Alabama State Department of Education.) *(continues)*

INDIVIDUALIZED EDUCATION PROGRAM

STUDENT'S NAME: _____

SPECIAL INSTRUCTIONAL FACTORS

Items checked "YES" will be addressed in this IEP:	YES	NO
• Does the student have behavior which impedes his/her learning or the learning of others?	[ ]	[ ]
• Does the student have limited English proficiency?	[ ]	[ ]
• Does the student need instruction in Braille and the use of Braille?	[ ]	[ ]
• Does the student have communication needs (deaf or hearing impaired only)?	[ ]	[ ]
• Does the student need assistive technology devices and/or services?	[ ]	[ ]
• Does the student require specially designed P.E.?	[ ]	[ ]
• Is the student working toward alternate achievement standards and participating in the Alabama Alternate Assessment?	[ ]	[ ]
• Are transition services addressed in this IEP?	[ ]	[ ]

TRANSPORTATION AS A RELATED SERVICE

Does the student require transportation as a related service?   [ ] YES [ ] NO

Does the student need accommodations or modifications for transportation?   [ ] YES [ ] NO

   If yes, check any transportation accommodations/modifications that are needed.

   [ ]   Bus driver is aware of student's behavioral and/or medical concerns

   [ ]   Wheelchair lift

   [ ]   Restraint system.
       Specify:

_____

   [ ]   Other.
       Specify:

_____

NONACADEMIC and EXTRACURRICULAR ACTIVITIES

Will the student have the opportunity to participate in nonacademic/extracurricular activities with his/her nondisabled peers?

   [ ]   YES.

   [ ]   YES, with supports. Describe:

_____

   [ ]   NO. Explanation must be provided:

_____

METHOD/FREQUENCY FOR REPORTING PROGRESS OF ATTAINING GOALS TO PARENTS

Annual Goal Progress reports will be sent to parents each time report cards are issued (every _____ weeks).

Page ____ of _____

SDE Approved 5/22/2007

Appendix L. *(continues)*

INDIVIDUALIZED EDUCATION PROGRAM

STUDENT'S NAME: _____

[ ] This student is in a middle school **course of study** that will help prepare him/her for transition.

EXIT OPTIONS (Complete for students in grades 9-12)

[ ] Alabama High School Diploma
    with Advanced Academic Endorsement

[ ] Alabama High School Diploma

[ ] Alabama Occupational Diploma

[ ] Graduation Certificate

[ ] Other _____

Anticipated Date of Exit:

_____   _____
Month   Year

PROGRAM CREDIT TO BE EARNED (Complete for students in grades 9-12)								
For each course taken, indicate program credit to be earned.	ENGLISH	MATH	SCIENCE	SOCIAL STUDIES				
Alabama High School Diploma with Advanced Academic Endorsement								
Alabama High School Diploma								
Alabama Occupational Diploma								
Graduation Certificate								

TRANSITION

(Beginning not later than the first IEP to be in effect when the student is 16,
or earlier if appropriate, and updated annually thereafter)

Transition Assessments (Check the assessment(s) used to determine the student's measurable transition goals):

[ ] Transition Planning Assessments   [ ] Interest Inventory   [ ] Other _____

Transition Goals:

Postsecondary Education/Employment Goal

_____

If **Other** is selected, specify

_____

Community/Independent Living Goal

_____

If **Other** is selected, specify

_____

Transition Services: **(Based on this student's strengths, preferences, and interests, the following coordinated transition services will reasonably enable the student to meet the postsecondary goals.)**

[ ] Vocational Evaluation (VE)
[ ] Employment Development (ED)
[ ] Postsecondary Education (PE)
[ ] Financial Management (FM)

[ ] Personal Management (PM)
[ ] Transportation (T)
[ ] Living Arrangements (LA)
[ ] Advocacy/Guardianship (AG)

[ ] Community Experiences (CE)
[ ] Medical (M)
[ ] Linkages to Agencies (L)
[ ] Other _____

TRANSFER OF RIGHTS

(Beginning not later than the IEP that will be in effect when the student reaches 18 years of age.)

Date student was informed that the rights under the IDEA will transfer to him/her at the age of 19 _____

SDE Approved 5/22/2007

Appendix L. *(continues)*

INDIVIDUALIZED EDUCATION PROGRAM

STUDENT'S NAME: _____

AREA: _____

PRESENT LEVEL OF ACADEMIC ACHIEVEMENT AND FUNCTIONAL PERFORMANCE:

MEASURABLE ANNUAL GOAL related to meeting the student's needs:

TYPE(S) OF EVALUATION FOR ANNUAL GOAL:

[ ] Curriculum Based Assessment [ ] Teacher/Text Test [ ] Teacher Observation [ ] Grades
[ ] Data Collection [ ] State Assessment(s) [ ] Work Samples
[ ] Other: _____
[ ] Other: _____

DATE OF MASTERY: _____

BENCHMARKS:
1.   Date of Mastery: _____
2.   Date of Mastery: _____
3.   Date of Mastery: _____
4.   Date of Mastery: _____

SPECIAL EDUCATION AND RELATED SERVICE(S): (Special Education, Supplementary Aids and Services, Program Modifications, Accommodations Needed for Assessments, Related Services, Assistive Technology, and Support for Personnel.)

Type of Service(s)	Anticipated Frequency of Service(s)	Amount of time	Beginning/ Ending Date	Location of Service(s)
Special Education			_____ to _____	
Supplementary Aids and Services			_____ to _____	
Program Modifications			_____ to _____	
Accommodations Needed for Assessments			_____ to _____	
Related Services			_____ to _____ _____ to _____	
Assistive Technology			_____ to _____	
Support for Personnel			_____ to _____	

Page _____ of _____

SDE Approved 5/22/007

Appendix L. *(continues)*

179

INDIVIDUALIZED EDUCATION PROGRAM

STUDENT'S NAME: _____

GENERAL FACTORS

HAS THE IEP TEAM CONSIDERED:	YES	NO
• The strengths of the child?	[ ]	[ ]
• The concerns of the parents for enhancing the education of the child?	[ ]	[ ]
• The results of the initial or most recent evaluations of the child?	[ ]	[ ]
• As appropriate, the results of performance on any State or districtwide assessments?	[ ]	[ ]
• The academic, developmental, and functional needs of the child?	[ ]	[ ]
• The need for extended school year services?	[ ]	[ ]

LEAST RESTRICTIVE ENVIRONMENT

Does this student attend the school (or for a preschool-age student, participate in the environment) he/she would attend if nondisabled?   [ ] Yes   [ ] No
If no, explain:

_____

Does this student receive all special education services with nondisabled peers? [ ] Yes [ ] No
If no, explain (explanation may not be solely because of needed modifications in the general curriculum):

_____

| | 6-21 YEARS OF AGE   [ ] 3-5 YEARS OF AGE
(Select one from the drop-down box.)

_____

Secondary LRE (only if LRE above is Private School-Parent Placed)

_____

COPY OF IEP

Was a copy of the IEP given to parent at the IEP meeting?
   [ ] Yes   [ ] No
If no, date sent to parent: _____

COPY OF *SPECIAL EDUCATION RIGHTS*

Was a copy of the *Special Education Rights* given to parent at the IEP meeting?   [ ] Yes   [ ] No
If no, date sent to parent: _____

Date copy of **amended** IEP provided/sent to parent _____

THE FOLLOWING PEOPLE ATTENDED AND PARTICIPATED IN THE MEETING TO DEVELOP THIS IEP.

Position	Signature	Date
Parent		
Parent		
LEA Representative		
Special Education Teacher		
General Education Teacher		
Student		
Career/Technical Education Rep		
Other Agency Representative		

INFORMATION FROM PEOPLE NOT IN ATTENDANCE

Position	Name	Date

Page _____ of _____

SDE Approved 5/22/007

Appendix L. *(continued)*

Example of an Annual Goal Progress Report Form Used in Public Schools

Annual Goal Progress Report

Student Name: _____

Student ID Number: _____

Date Sent: _____

IEP Initiation/Duration Dates From: _____ to _____

School Year: _____

IEP Annual Review Date: _____

Use the legends below to evaluate the student's progress toward the annual goals. The 1st column should indicate the *Report of Progress* using the numbers 1-4. The 2nd column should indicate the *Extent of Progress* using the numbers 1-4.

Report of Progress on Annual Goals
1. Goal has been met.
2. Some progress made.
3. Very little progress made.
4. No progress made.

Extent of Progress Toward Meeting the Annual Goals
1. Goal mastered.
2. Anticipate mastery.
3. Do not anticipate mastery.
4. *NA* Not applicable during this grading period.

Report/Extent of Progress

Record Date of Reporting Periods

Measurable Annual Goals

School System
School Name

6/1/2006

Appendix M. Example of an Annual Goal Progress Report Form Used in Public Schools. (Used with permission from Alabama State Department of Education.)

Example of a University Clinic Long-Term Treatment Report

TREATMENT REPORT

Name: John Smith   **File Number:** 00-345-0

Age: 15   **D.O.B.:** 1-20-93

Address: 1234 Oak St.
Anytown, USA

Date of Report: 5-1-08   **Phone Number:** 334-123-4567

Clinician: K. Gates   **Period Covered:** Spring 2008

Number of Sessions Attended: 12 out of 12 scheduled sessions

Scheduled Sessions: 60 minutes 1 time per week

Current Background Information

John is a 15-year-old male who is in the ninth grade in a regular classroom. He was evaluated at this clinic on October 1, 2007. According to the Stuttering Severity Instrument (SSI-3), he exhibits a moderate to severe fluency disorder, which has a significant impact on his daily interactions. John was receiving speech therapy through the public schools, but was referred to this clinic for further assessment and treatment.

Current Evaluation Results

Date of Evaluation: October 1, 2007

Assessment Tool: Stuttering Severity Instrument (SSI-3)

Results:

    Total Score: 34

    Percentile rank: 89–95%

    Severity rating: Severe

Assessment of the Child's Experience of Stuttering (ACES)

    Total Impact Score: 61 (Moderate to Severe)

    Reports most difficulty with ordering food, telling stories, asking a question in class

Objectives and Progress

LTG 1: The client will achieve a comfortable level of fluency at the conversational level in social and academic settings.

STO A: The client will utilize a smooth and easy rate during structured reading tasks on 4/5 opportunities.

    Baseline Data: 2-7-08   22% dysfluent

    Final Data: 2-28-08   6% dysfluent

Materials: Eight- to 10-words sentences from *HELP* workbook

Cues: Clinician models smooth rate; "Remember to smooth out your speech."

Reinforcement: Verbal praise, replay audio tape

STO B: The client will utilize smooth and easy speech during structured conversation in order to decrease dysfluencies to less than 10% during a 60-minute session.

    Baseline Data: 2-28-08   31% dysfluent

    Final Data: 4-18-08   18% dysfluent

Materials: "Guess Who," "Conversation," spontaneous conversation with clinician

Cues: Verbal cue to remind him of his "speech rules"

Reinforcement: Verbal praise, "I like how you said that," "Very smooth speech"

STO C: The client will utilize the Easy Onset technique during a structured reading task with 90% accuracy.

    Baseline Data: 3-14-08   10% accuracy

    Final Data: 3-28-08   80% accuracy

Materials: Short paragraphs from *The Source for Aphasia Therapy* workbook

Cues: "Remember to ease into the first word," clinician models technique

Reinforcement: Replay video tape, verbal praise

STO D: The client will utilize the Easy Onset technique when having difficulty initiating spontaneous speech on 4/5 communication opportunities.

    Baseline Data: 3-28-08   0 times

    Final Data: 4-18-08   4/10 times

Materials: None

Cues: "It sounded like you had difficulty with the word _____," "Let's try that again," clinician models technique

Summary/Recommendations

John made great progress this semester regarding his awareness of moments of dysfluency, as well as identifying which strategies were most helpful for him. Even though he initially reported that his stuttering does not hold him back in any way, he eventually shared with the clinician that he sometimes avoided certain speaking situations. With increased confidence regarding use of his techniques, John has a more positive attitude regarding his speech and stated that he felt therapy had been very helpful for him. It is recommended that John continue with speech therapy at the A.U. Speech and Hearing clinic at a frequency of 1 time per week for 60-minute sessions during the fall semester. Treatment goals should focus on:

1. Increased awareness of moments of stuttering and avoidance techniques
2. Increasing the client's efficiency in using fluency shaping techniques (Easy Onset)
3. Improving fluency in unstructured speaking situations

Example of Discharge Summary from Rehabilitation Hospital

REGIONAL
Rehabilitation Hospital

A JOINT VENTURE BETWEEN COLUMBUS REGIONAL AND HEALTHSOUTH

DATE ___/___/___   ☐ DISCHARGE SUMMARY

Documentation should include:Barriers to Discharge including Safety,
Bowel & Bladder, Mood & Behavior, and Nutrition/Hydration as they impact Therapy

PHYSICAL THERAPY	FUNCTIONAL LEVEL	DEVICE	PROGRESS SUMMARY/GOALS MET
BED MOBILITY			
AMBULATION			
W/C MOBILITY			
BALANCE			
SITTING			
STANDING			
STAIRS			NEW WEEKLY GOALS/DISCHARGE STATUS
CURBS			
TRANSFERS			
			EDUCATION
			PAIN MANAGEMENT

SIGNATURE(s):

OCCUPATIONAL THERAPY	FUNCTIONAL LEVEL	DEVICE	PROGRESS SUMMARY/GOALS MET
EATING			
GROOMING			
DRESSING-UE			
DRESSING-LE			
BATHING			
TOILETING			NEW WEEKLY GOALS/DISCHARGE STATUS
IADLs			
TRANSFERS			
			EDUCATION
			PAIN MANAGEMENT

SIGNATURE(s):

SPEECH THERAPY	FUNCTIONAL LEVEL	PROGRESS SUMMARY/GOALS MET
COMPREHENSION		
EXPRESSION		
INTELLIGIBILITY		
MEMORY		NEW WEEKLY GOALS/DISCHARGE STATUS
ATTENTION		
PROBLEM SOLVING		
SWALLOWING		
		EDUCATION
		PAIN MANAGEMENT

SIGNATURE(s):

Updated: 01/03/05   103a-PT,OT,SP Weekly Note

Appendix O. Example of a Discharge Summary from Rehabilitation Hospital. (Used with permission from Healthsouth Corporation.)

Example of a Long-Term Care Facility Progress Note

SPEECH/LANGUAGE-DYSPHAGIA WEEKLY PROGRESS NOTE

☐ Weekly Note ☐ Discharge Summary   Service Dates: _____ to _____

Check all that apply: ☐ Aphasia ☐ Dysphagia ☐ Cognitive Deficits ☐ Symbolic Language Dysfunction ☐ Motor Speech ☐ Aural Rehab Other:

Abbreviated Goals	Baseline (Initial & DC)	Previous Week	Current Week

Skilled Services: - Diagnostic treatment -Type and level of cues -Stimulus material -Equipment recommended -Analysis/effectiveness of compensatory strategies -Treatment plan modifications -Additional information **Group Therapy** - Provided this week: ☐ Yes ☐ No If yes, # of participants, activities performed, goal(s) addressed

Functional Outcomes: -Progress that positively affects quality of life   -Response to treatment -Patient's response to caregiver's use of strategies

Caregiver Education: -Person being trained -Type of training/education - Caregiver's return demonstration

Comments/justification for continued skilled services (i.e., functional problems remaining, positive potential for reaching goals, reasons for limited progress, etc.)

COMPLETE AT DISCHARGE	Last treatment completion time:	Visits from SOC:	FMP Program ☐ yes ☐ no

Discharge to: ☐ Restorative Nurse ☐ Nursing ☐ Hospital ☐ Home ☐ Assisted Living ☐ Expired ☐ Other: _____

Functional Outcome Scale: 0=Dependent 1=Severe 2=Mod. Severe 3=Mod 4=Mod. Mild 5=Mild 6=Independent

Auditory Comprehension:___ Verbal Expression:___ Cognition:___ Non-Verbal:___ Intelligibility:____Dysphagia:____ Oral:___ Pharyngeal:___ Liquid:___ Solid:___

Therapist Signature: _____   Date: _____

Room #:	Patient #:	Patient Name:	Facility:	Physician:

RT-110A   5/30/05

Appendix P. Example of a Long-Term Care Facility Progress Note. (Used with Permission from Restore Therapy.)

Example of a Discharge Summary from an Acute Care Hospital

BAYVIEW HOSPITAL

Patient Name: Jane Doe   **DOB/Age/Sex:** 3/21/31   77 Years Female

Admitting Physician: Jones

Admission Date: 7/17/08

Speech Discharge Summary

7/25/08   4:30 p.m.   Performed by: John Smith, SLP

Goals

Speech/Language/Patient/Caregiver Goals: Goals not met as progress has not been made.

Speech/Language Goal

1—Pt. will follow multi-step commands with 80% accuracy with no cueing required.

2—Pt. will answer complex y/n questions with 80% accuracy.

3—Pt. will answer questions regarding paragraphs read aloud with 80% accuracy.

4—Pt. will answer questions regarding orientation to time and place with 80% accuracy.

Baseline:

1—2/3 two-step commands

2—3/5 y/n questions

3—2/3 simple y/n questions

4—Place: 1/3

   Time: 1/4

ST Discharge Summary: Pt. is being discharged at this time as no progress has been made with current goals following evaluation. Patient is at prior level of function. Three day trial therapy completed today.

References

Alabama State Department of Education. (n.d.). *Mastering the maze*. Retrieved December 23, 2007, from http://www.alsde.edu

American Academy of Pediatrics. (2007). Professionalism in pediatrics. *Pediatrics, 120*(4), 895–897.

American Speech-Language-Hearing Association (ASHA). (2004). Retrieved April 26, 2007, from http://www.asha.org/members/ebp/default

American Speech-Language-Hearing Association (ASHA). (2003). ASHA Code of Ethics. Retrieved November 7, 2007, from http://www.asha.org/NR/rdonlyres/F51E46C5-3D87-44AF-BFDA-346D32F85C60/0/v1CodeOfEthics.pdf

American Speech-Language-Hearing Association. (2004). Paul, D. (1994), updated by Hasselkus, A. (2004). *Clinical record keeping in speech-language pathology for health care and third-party payers.*

ASHA Committee on Supervision. (1985). Clinical supervision in speech-language pathology, *ASHA, 27*, 57–60.

Anderson, J. (1988). *The supervisory process in speech-language pathology and audiology*. Austin, TX: Pro-Ed.

Battle, D. (1997). Multicultural considerations in counseling communicatively disordered persons and their families. In T. Crowe (Ed.), *Applications of counseling in speech-language pathology and audiology* (pp. 118–144). Baltimore: Williams & Wilkins.

Boone, D., McFarlane, S., & Von Berg, S. (2005). *The voice and voice therapy*. Needham Heights, MA: Allyn & Bacon.

Brehm, B., Breen, P., Brown, B., Long, L., Smith, R., Wall, A., et al. (2006). An interdisciplinary approach to introducing professionalism. *American Journal of Pharmaceutical Education, 70*(4), 1–5, Article 81.

Brown, R. (1973). *A first language: The early stages*. Boston: Harvard University Press.

Centers for Medicare and Medicaid Services (CMS). Retrieved February 2, 2008, from http://www.cms.hhs.gov

Clooman, P., Davis, F., & Burnett, C. (1999). Interdisciplinary education in clinical ethics: A work in progress. *Holistic Nursing Practice, 13*, 9–12.

Consumer Driven Health Care. (n.d.). *Glossary definition of third party payment*. Retrieved May 2, 2008, from http://cdhc.ncpa.org

Council of Exceptional Children (CEC). Retrieved January 23, 2008, from http://www.cec.sped.org

Crowe, T. (1997). *Applications of counseling in speech-language pathology and audiology*. Baltimore: Williams & Wilkins.

Damico, J. (1987). Addressing language concerns in the schools: The SLP as consultant. *Journal of Childhood Communication Disorders, 11*, 17–40.

Emerick, L. (1969). *The parent interview*. Danville, IL: Interstate.

Family Educational Rights and Privacy Act (FERPA). Retrieved July 5, 2008, from http://www.ed.gov/policy/gen/guid/fpco/ferpa/index.html

Ferguson, M. (1991). Collaborative/consultative service delivery: An introduction. *Language, Speech and Hearing Services in Schools, 22*, 147.

Frassinelli, L., Superior, K., & Meyers, J. (1983). A consultation model for speech and language intervention. *Journal of the American Speech-Language-Hearing Association, 25*(11), 25–30.

French, S., & Sim, J. (1993). *Writing: A guide for therapists*. Oxford, UK: Butterworth-Heineman.

Fujiki, M., & Brinton, B. (1984). Supplementing language therapy: Working with the classroom teachers. *Language, Speech and Hearing Services in Schools, 15*, 98–109.

Gregory, H. (2003). *Stuttering therapy: Rationale and procedures*. Needham Heights, MA: Allyn & Bacon.

Hammer, D., Berger, B., & Beardsley, R. (2003). Student professionalism. *American Journal of Pharmaceutical Education, 67*, 1–29.

Hasselkus, A., & Paul, D. (2004). Retrieved April 22, 2008, from http://www.asha.org

Haynes, W., & Hartman, D. (1975). The agony of report writing: A new look at an old problem. *Journal of the National Student Speech and Hearing Association, 3*, 7–15.

Haynes, W., & Johnson, C. (2009). *Understanding research and evidence-based practice in communication disorders: A primer for students and practitioners.* Boston: Allyn & Bacon.

Haynes, W., Moran, M., & Pindzola, R. (2006). *Communication disorders in the classroom* (4th ed.). Boston: Jones & Bartlett.

Haynes, W., & Pindzola, R. (2008). *Diagnosis and evaluation in speech pathology* (7th ed.). Boston: Allyn & Bacon.

Health Information Portability and Accountability Act (HIPAA). Retrieved July 8, 2008, from http://www.hhs.gov/ocr/hipaa/

Hegde, M., & Davis, D. (1995). *Clinical methods and practicum in speech-language pathology* (2nd ed.). San Diego, CA: Singular.

Individuals with Disabilities Education Act. (IDEA, 2004). (IDEA Part C and Related Topics). Retrieved October 15, 2007, from http://www.ideapartnership.org/topicdetail.cfm?topicid=33

Klein, H., & Moses, N. (1994). *Intervention planning for children with communication disorders: A guide for clinical practicum and professional practice.* Englewood Cliffs, NJ: Prentice-Hall.

Knepflar, K. (1976). Report writing for private practitioners. In R. Battin & D. Fox (Eds.), *Private practice in audiology and speech pathology* (pp. 115–136). New York: Grune and Stratton.

Locke, J. L. (1980). The inference of speech perception in the phonologically disordered child. Part I. A rationale, some criteria, the conventional tests. *Journal of Speech and Hearing Disorders, 40*, 431–444.

Magnotta, O. (1991). Looking beyond tradition. *Language, Speech and Hearing Services in Schools, 22*, 150–151.

Marvin, C. (1987). Consultation services: Changing roles for SLPs. *Journal of Childhood Communication Disorders, 11*(1), 1–16.

Matarazzo, J., & Wiens, A. (1972). *The interview: Research on its anatomy and structure.* Chicago: Aldine-Atherton.

McQuire, M., & Lorch, S. (1968). A model for the study of dyadic communication. *Journal of Nervous and Mental Disease, 146*, 221–229.

Medfriendly. (2008). *Uniform data system for medical rehabilitation.* Retrieved February 9, 2008, from http://www.medfriendly.com/functionalindependencemeasure.html

Meitus, I. (1983). Clinical report and letter writing. In I. Meitus & B. Weinberg (Eds.), *Diagnosis in speech-language pathology* (pp. 287–307). Baltimore: University Park Press.

Meyer, S. (2004). *Survival guide for the beginning speech-language pathologist* (2nd ed.). Austin, TX: Pro-Ed.

Middleton, G., Pannbacker, M., Vekovius, G. T., Sanders, K. L., & Pluett, V. (1992). *Report writing for speech-language pathologists.* Tuscon, AZ: Communication Skill Builders.

Miller, R. & Groher, M. (1990). *Medical speech pathology.* Gaithersburg, MD: Aspen.

Montgomery, J. (1992). Implementing collaborative consultation: Perspectives from the field. *Language, Speech and Hearing Services in Schools, 23*, 363–364.

Moon-Meyer, S, (2004). *Survival guide for the beginning speech-language clinician.* Austin, TX: Pro-Ed.

Moore, M. (1969). Pathological writing. *ASHA, 11*, 535–538.

Moore-Brown, B. (1991). Moving in the direction of change: Thoughts for administrators and speech-language pathologists. *Language, Speech and Hearing Services in Schools, 22*, 148–149.

National Dissemination Center for Children and Youth with Disabilities. (2008). Retrieved August 28, 2008 from http://www.nichey.org

Nebraska Department of Education. (n.d.). *Measurable annual goals, benchmarks and short-term objectives: What are they?* Retrieved January 4, 2008, from http://www.nde.state.ne.us/SPED/iepproj/develop/mea.html

Nelson. (1973). Structure and strategy in learning to talk. *Monographs of the Society for Research in Child Development, 38*, 11–56.

Nelson, K. E., Camarata, S. M., Welsh, J. Butkovsky, L. & Camarata, M. (1996). Effects of imitative and conversational recasting treatment on the acquisition of grammar in children with specific language impairment and younger language-normal children. *Journal of Speech and Hearing Research, 39*, 850–859.

Owens, R., Metz, D., & Haas, A. (2000). *Introduction to communication disorders: A life span perspective.* Needham Heights, MA: Allyn & Bacon.

Packer, B. (1995). *Improving writing skills in SLP graduate students through a clinical writing course.* Davie, FL: Nova University ERIC.

Pannbacker, M., Middleton, G., Vekovius, G., & Sanders, K. (2001). *Report writing for speech-language pathologists*. Austin, TX: Communication Skill Builders.

Paul. (2001). Language Disorders from Infancy through Adolescence. St. Louis: Mosby.

Randolph, D. (2003). Evaluating the professional behaviors of entry-level occupational therapy students. *Journal of Allied Health, 32*, 116–121.

Roseberry-McKibbin, C. (1997). Working with linguistically and culturally diverse clients. In K. Shipley (Ed.), *Interviewing and counseling in communicative disorders: Principles and procedures* (pp. 151–172). Boston: Allyn & Bacon.

Shipley, K. (1997). *Interviewing and counseling in communicative disorders: Principles and procedures.* Boston: Allyn & Bacon.

Shipley, K., & McAfee, J. (1998). *Assessment in speech-language pathology: A resource manual* (2nd ed.). San Diego, CA: Singular-Thomson Learning.

Smit, A. B., Hand, L., Freilinger, J., Bernthal, J., & Bird, A. (1990). The Iowa articulation norms project and its Nebraska reduplication. *Journal of Speech and Hearing Disorders, 55*, 779–798.

Stewart, C., & Cash, W. (1974). *Interviewing: Principles and practices*. Dubuque, IA: W. C. Brown.

Strunk, W., & White, E. B. (2000). *The elements of style* (4th ed.). Needham Heights, MA: Allyn & Bacon.

United States Department of Education. (2005). *A guide to the Individualized Education Program.* Retrieved October 12, 2006, from http://www.ed.gov/parents/needs/speced/iepguide/index.html

Van Riper, C., & Emerick, L. (1984). *Speech correction: An introduction to speech pathology and audiology.* Englewood Cliffs, NJ: Prentice-Hall.

Yarrus, S. (2007, November). *Practical treatment strategies for preschool and school-age children who stutter.* Paper presented at the convention of the American Speech-Language-Hearing Association, Boston, MA.

Zinsser, W. K. (2006). *On writing well.* New York: Harper Collins.

Index